HEALED, HEALTHY AND WHOLE

How We Beat Cancer with Integrated
Therapies and Essential Healing Strategies

MARION M. PYLE

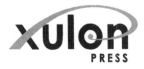

Healed, Healthy and Whole
How We Beat Cancer with Integrated Therapies and Essential Healing Strategies
by Marion M. Pyle

Printed in the United States of America

ISBN 9781629520988

Unless otherwise indicated, Bible quotations are taken from Zondervan NIV Study Bible. Copyright © 2008 by Kenneth L. Baker.

Spring, Fall, Winter, Concluding Thoughts, Scripture Verses photos by Marion M. Pyle. Light Echo around V838 Monocerotis by NASA, ESA, and the Hubble Heritage Team (STSc/AURA)

www.xulonpress.com

DEDICATION

This book is lovingly dedicated to...

Almighty God, the Father, Son and Holy Spirit
— Who, in a mighty, merciful and unforgettable descent,
taught these two ragamuffins how to walk on water.

My precious husband, Russell.
You are the song in my heart and the love of my life.

Our family, Christian family, pastors, and friends.
It will take more than this lifetime to express our gratitude
for the joy and privilege of your love,
faithfulness and friendship.

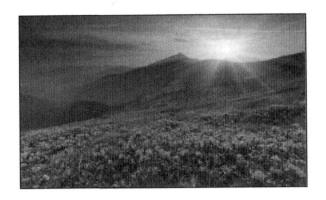

Jesus, draw me ever nearer
as I labor through the storm.
You have called me to this passage,
and I'll follow, though I'm worn.
May this journey bring a blessing,
may I rise on wings of faith.
And at the end of my heart's testing,
with Your likeness let me wake.
Jesus, guide me through the tempest,
keep my spirit staid and sure.
When the midnight meets the morning,
let me love You even more.
Let the treasures of the trial
form within me as I go.
And at the end of this long passage,
let me leave them at Your throne.

- Keith Getty and Margaret Becker

TABLE OF CONTENTS

PART III: FALL

PART IV: WINTER

PART V: CONCLUDING THOUGHTS

PART VI: ADDITIONAL RESOURCES

Preface

Blessed are those whose strength is in You, who have set their hearts on pilgrimage.
As they pass through the Valley of Baca,* they make it a place of springs;
the autumn rains also cover it with pools.
They go from strength to strength, till each appears before God in Zion.
— Psalm 84:5-7

* From the Hebrew word *bakah*,
meaning "to weep, bewail or shed tears."

On a sunny day in March 2012, my husband and love of my life, Russell, was diagnosed with malevolent bladder cancer. It was the worst kind; so bad, in fact, it would not even respond to chemotherapy. The doctors were 95-percent sure they'd have to take his bladder out to save his life. However, ten months later Russell's cancer was gone without a trace. Today, he is healed, healthy and his bladder is whole and intact!

What made this possible? Was it the integrative therapies? The diet and nutrition? Was it our faith? The blanket of prayers? Was it a combination of these? Or was it quite simply... a miracle?

One thing we do know: Our experience with cancer has so radically transformed our lives that today we feel passionate about sharing with others the strategies, resources and insights that helped heal and preserve Russell's life—and mine, too, for to see a loved one attacked by a hideous disease is to also suffer a terrible agony.

Among the many approaches we explain, you will find integrative therapies (the combination of mainstream medical treatments with non-toxic, non-invasive natural therapies) that are proving successful in overcoming many kinds of cancers, as well as other chronic illnesses. These are exciting and encouraging discoveries.

It is worth stating that I do not benefit financially from any of the resources listed in this book. I share them simply because they benefited us greatly.

Neither am I a doctor or integrative specialist; the combination of treatments we followed were the result of our own research, education, and prayerful consideration, as well as consultations with many medical and alternative therapy professionals. Our approach should not be mistaken for a prescriptive one-size-fits-all formula for someone else's illness or condition. Healing approaches must be tailored to each person's individual needs in step with the recommendations of doctors and specialists of their choice.

However, we do believe that our discoveries can raise positive awareness about the world of integrative therapies and the multiple benefits available to those battling many kinds of common cancers and other chronic conditions.

In the beginning, we knew none of these things. Our journey was terrifying, painful and difficult. That's what made our recovery all the more stunning. To us, our story does seem like a special miracle; one we celebrate and thank God for every day.

We're also clear that our journey was not just about us. We are now committed to helping others also find physical, emotional and spiritual wellness. We know that we were blessed to be a blessing. And so, in that spirit, this book is an offering to all who are searching. We pray it not only provides the hope, guidance and resources you need, but that one day you and your loved one are also able to say, "I am healed, healthy and whole."

Introduction

Gratitude makes sense of our past, brings peace for today,

and creates a vision for tomorrow.

—Melody Beattie

The Enigma

According to the American Cancer Society, nine out of every 10 bladder-cancer victims is over the age of 55. Russell fits this category.

But, in other ways, he was a most unlikely candidate. Russ had always lived a healthy lifestyle. He ate wholesome foods and exercised regularly. He didn't smoke or abuse alcohol. He was fit and vigorous. It was unimaginable that he should fall prey to cancer. In fact, friends said the words 'Russell' and 'cancer' didn't even fit in the same sentence.

The World of Us

In 2012, Russell and I were living in Los Angeles, California. We had been married 15 years, and for both of us, they had been the happiest of our lives. We shared a passion for the our faith, the arts, media and entertainment; and we'd both worked and served in various facets of these industries since we were young.

His Story

Russell was Pasadena-born and raised, and had lived in Southern California pretty much his entire life. Over the years, he'd established himself as a daring, innovative and award-winning set-and-lighting designer. His work took him all over the world, and fed his love of adventure and other cultures.

In fact, as a ministry, Russell enjoyed smuggling Bibles into restricted countries throughout Asia. He was so fearless, I nicknamed him "Indy," after Indiana Jones. We'd joke that me joining him on these missions trips had been a prenuptial condition!

And we did indeed partner on many risky journeys to China, North and South Vietnam, to refugee camps on the Thai/Burma border, and to Cambodia. They were all wonderful, enriching experiences (topics for another book)!

My Story

My story began in Buenos Aires, Argentina, where I was born to Scottish-American parents. My father was a television executive for a U.S. broadcast network. When I was six, he was transferred to Mexico City to head operations for Latin America.

Our home was often filled with American producers, directors and actors, and screenings of the latest U.S. television series. I frequently accompanied my father to the Hollywood studios, and would watch, enthralled, as many of everyone's favorite shows came to life.

It was a foregone conclusion that I'd also go into "the biz," as people in the entertainment industry call it. This path took me from Mexico to Los Angeles, and later Melbourne, Australia.

My passion was acting, but over the years, I also wrote, produced and directed for theater and television, as well as doing stints in advertising. While living in Melbourne, I also co-founded a boutique drama studio that became a creative home to many wonderful artists. To this day, it holds a special place in my heart.

Transformational Encounters

My time in Australia was also memorable in another sense: It was here that I found God and became a Christian. (Well, the way it really works is that God finds *you* and then your life's real purpose comes into focus.)

My transformation awakened a voracious spiritual thirst that drove me to Bible college. After completing my studies, God distinctly called me back to Los Angeles.

Sometime after my return, I volunteered at a Thanksgiving dinner that serves homeless families in Santa Monica, California. A man named Russell Pyle was one of the leaders, and I was assigned to work with him for the day. As he tells it, I made quite an impression.

Swept Up

One thing led to another and we started dating. Now, Russell is a true romantic, and over the ensuing months he wooed me with moonlit horseback rides, personally cooked gourmet meals, spectacular surprise birthday parties, touching poetry, and more! (Yes, topics for another book!)

The Big Moment

It all culminated one summer evening at Zuma Beach in Malibu. As our limo pulled up, there in the distance, against the setting sun, stood a table for two dressed with dazzling white linen, crystal candleholders, fine china, and French champagne on ice. The beach was empty, as if God had reserved it just for us.

An exquisite dinner was waiting in silver chafing dishes. Russell had personally prepared everything earlier in the day. He'd also instructed two of his friends about how to set the table and accessories, so it looked stunning for when we arrived in our limo at 7 o'clock.

As my eyes took in this breathtaking scene, the purpose of the evening became patently obvious. The surprise was so overwhelming, I was sure that the thunder of my pounding heart would upstage the conversation!

After our exquisite meal, as the sun was slowly setting, Russ asked me to close my eyes and take off my shoes. What followed was not just unexpected, but took my breath away. When I was finally able to open my eyes, I found him kneeling on the sand in front of me. Gently taking my bare feet, he washed them in a tub of warm water. After carefully toweling them dry, he looked up at me with his big baby blues and, smiling, said:

"I want to honor, serve and love you all the days of my life. Will you be my wife?"

What do *you* think I said!?

Moving into the Present

Moving ahead to the present brings us to the time of this story. Russell was busy working as a technical producer, editor and audiovisual guru. I'd just completed my eighth and final season as writer, producer and co-host of a cable television show and was exploring an opportunity in public relations.

A Rude Awakening

The sudden cancer diagnosis completely rocked our world. It felt like being ambushed—and a case could certainly be made for that, in spiritual terms.

Our journey took a little over 10 months. It was a heart-wrenching, terrifying ride into the unknown. We had breakthroughs and letdowns, advances and set-backs, good news and dashed hopes... but we never gave up.

Those of you who *have* been there—or are there *now*—know how life gets stripped down to the most vital essentials as you laser focus on healing and sur-vival. Yet through the terror and confusion, God began working good out of this evil every step of the way. It strengthened our marriage, deepened our faith, enriched our friendships, and birthed a new ministry.

Family and friends reported that it brought *them* closer to God as well, and also awakened a new awareness of the power of prayer and the spiritual dimension behind every aspect of their lives.

A Tribute, Blessing, and Thank You

In these next chapters, you will find the spiritual, nutritional and integrative strategies that contributed to Russell's ultimate healing. We offer them for three important reasons:

1. As a tribute to God, who knew before the beginning of time that we would walk through this "valley of the shadow of death" (Psalm 23:4), and pre-pared the way with such an unforgettable display of love, grace and mercy that it must be shouted from the rooftops.
2. As an offering to our readers, with hope that something in our story may help you or your loved one find health, healing and wholeness.

3. As a "thank you" to the dozens of family members, friends, doctors, pastors, ministry leaders, and counselors who stood by us in our hour of need, with a loyalty and devotion that strengthened our feeble knees and taught us the splendor and power of community. We would not have made it through without the extraordinary support of this precious group of people.

So, without further ado, this is our story. May it richly bless you as you journey through its pages.

> **Declare His glory among the nations, His marvelous deeds among all peoples.**
> **—Psalm 96:3**

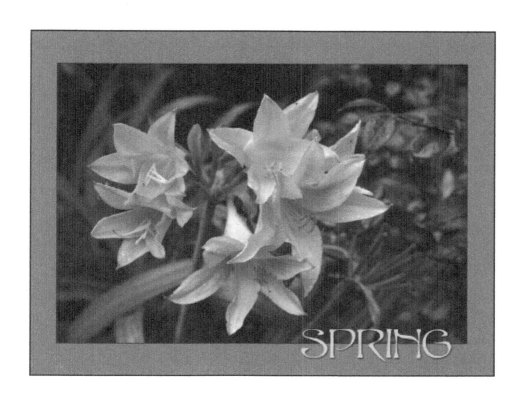

CHAPTER 1
A SUDDEN SHIFT IN THE WIND

Life can only be understood backwards;
but it must be lived forwards.
— Søren Kierkegaard

Our journey began when I was working as a vice president at a prestigious public-relations firm. Our country's economic crunch was beginning to take its toll and we were feeling it at the office.

Clients were bailing and budgets were shrinking. Then, the sudden and untimely death of the company president shook the firm to its foundations and stripped it of a luminous leader.

A few months later, we were informed this independent company was being sold to a global giant. Within a few weeks, together with several others, I was laid off.

The news was not entirely unexpected and, actually, turned out to be a blessing in disguise. For more than two and a half years, the stress, long hours and killer commute had been impacting my marriage and my health. I had become increasingly unhappy, restless and longed for more creative pursuits. Now, the decision had been made for me and a huge weight had lifted off my shoulders.

Home Sweet Home

I would now be able to work from my home office until I could regroup and discern my next move. I couldn't wait to focus on several personal writing and producing projects that had been sitting on the back burner for years. The prospect of resurrecting these was thrilling.

I felt the wind under my wings and optimism in my heart.

I was also absolutely clueless about what awaited Russell and me around the bend.

CHAPTER 2
The Ambush

The thief comes only to steal, kill and destroy.
— Jesus, in John 10:10

I t was an evening in March when Russell suddenly noticed blood in his urine. Perplexed, we did some research and learned that bleeding is not uncommon among athletes. Since Russ followed a rigorous daily exercise regime, we thought nothing of it.

Well, let me rephrase that: *I* thought nothing of it.

Russell, the born optimist, was uncharacteristically worried. Being a fitness enthusiast, he was in great shape and highly sensitive to any imbalances in his body.

At first, we thought the bleeding would just stop, but the episodes recurred. Wanting to comfort him, I assured Russell it was most likely a torn muscle or ligament—and I honestly believed it. Russ was a strong and healthy man.

But when the bleeding reappeared over the next two, then three weeks, our family doctor urged Russell to see a specialist.

It took two months of consultations and tests before the day finally came to get the final results.

CHAPTER 3
A HIDEOUS INTRUDER

Courage is grace under pressure.

— Ernest Hemingway

It was Wednesday afternoon, June 7th. We found ourselves in a well-known urologist's office. Outside the window, sparrows chirped brightly in the pine trees. The antiseptic room was bathed in soft sunlight.

It was four o'clock.

"Your urine tested positive for high-grade bladder cancer," the urologist announced matter-of-factly.

Our hearts stopped.

"What?" I asked, completely shocked. "Could you repeat that?"

The urologist looked down at his report.

"The diagnosis is high-grade urothelial carcinoma."

Time stood still.

"I knew it was cancer," Russell said in a whisper.

I fell back in my chair, speechless.

"We need to do an exam," said the doctor, patting the long table next to him. "Please come up here."

Russell readied himself and lay flat. A black, 20-inch monitor was suspended directly above him. The doctor then took a slender tube; its tip held a small light and video camera. The doctor inserted it through the opening in Russell's urethra, moving up inside until the tip reached Russell's bladder.

Though it was obviously unpleasant and uncomfortable, Russ said it wasn't actually "painful."

As the probe journeyed upward, the monitor clearly displayed Russell's clean and pink internal tissues. It felt surreal to see his insides as clearly as we could see the exterior world around us.

When the probe finally reached the bladder, the doctor announced: "There's the tumor."

The monitor revealed a small, bloody mass about half of an inch in size; it looked like it had erupted from otherwise healthy, pink bladder tissue.

"Can you see it?" the doctor asked.

"Yes," I whispered, my heart pounding. I felt a sense of outrage at this hideous intruder that threatened our happy life.

"This should come out right away," announced the doctor. "Are you available next week?"

Russell nodded.

And so it began. In the blink of an eye, we were catapulted from our peaceful world into "the valley of the shadow of death" (Psalm 23:4).

Russell picked up his phone. Then, swiping through his calendar, he forwarded to Wednesday, June 13—exactly one week away—and blocked out the entire day. Steadying his trembling fingers, he typed in: "Surgery... for cancer."

CHAPTER 4
SHAKEN TO THE CORE

Prayer is not believing in my own unshakable belief.
Faith is believing in an unshakable God
when everything in me trembles and quakes.
— Beth Moore

The week leading up to the surgery was torture. Had we caught the cancer early? Had it spread to other organs? Had Russell only a few weeks to live? Our minds wrestled with a thousand questions: What if... what then... what now?

Russell was quiet and pensive, but expressed faith that things would turn out well.

I put on a brave face, but trembled inside in places I did not know could quake. Having lost my mother in an airplane accident at the age of 12—one of several devastating losses throughout my life—the prospect of now losing Russell, my best friend, my lover and life companion, triggered the deepest, most-terrible fear.

> **You of little faith, why are you so afraid?**
> **—Jesus, in Matthew 8:26**

I'd been a woman of prayer for 25 years. Intercessory prayer (praying fervently for the needs of others on their behalf) was one of my strongest ministries. I'd experienced and witnessed hundreds, or probably thousands, of inspiring and miraculous answers to prayer over the years. But this cancer hit so close to home, I was shaken to the core.

Lord, Take My Hand

Wherever you land on the theological spectrum—that is, whether you believe God sovereignly shapes trials to help us mature (even those calamities that bring us to our knees), or that attacks come from the enemy of our souls—one still has to get through them. And the *only* way is to admit to God that you are helpless and terrified, and that you desperately need Him to guide you through the unknown.

CHAPTER 5
KISSED BY GRACE

**Do not be anxious about anything, but in every situation, by prayer
and petition, with thanksgiving, present your requests to God. And
the peace of God, which transcends all understanding, will guard your
hearts and minds in Christ Jesus.**
— Philippians 4:6-7

On Wednesday, June 13 at 7 a.m., Russell and I checked into the hospital. We walked through a beige-colored lobby corridor flanked by soft watercolors. We took the elevator to the third-floor waiting area.

Floor-to-ceiling windows flooded the spacious waiting area with morning light. A few families had already settled into a few of the armchairs and sofas; they were speaking in hushed tones.

Despite our anxiety, the environment was peaceful.

Friends in Time of Need

Two members of our Christian home group arose to greet us: Carmen, a chaplain, and Janet, a playwright. They were both dear friends—what a comfort it was to have them there!

We settled into a quiet nook. We clasped hands and prayed, asking God to guide all the events of the day and to give the doctors wisdom and skill.

The memories of all the previous times I'd accompanied loved ones to the hospital came flooding back. I clung to Jesus for strength.

Life's Fragile Thread

Carmen brought us a Health Care Directive to fill out. Also called an "advance directive" or "living will," this legal document allowed Russell to appoint me as his agent, so I could make healthcare decisions for him should he become incapacitated. It was a sober reminder of life's fragile thread.

Russ and I then stepped into an office to finalize admittance papers.

On the right corner of the desk, the following Bible verse was displayed in a small frame:

> **May the God of hope fill you with all joy and peace as you trust in Him.**
> **— Romans 15:13**

I smiled to myself and exhaled deeply.

Suddenly, the admissions nurse, a complete stranger, looked at Russell and said: "God wants me to tell you that you are going to be all right."

Our jaws dropped.

"Wow—thank you!" laughed Russell.

Then, turning to me she said: "You both needed to hear that."

"We certainly did!" I said, stunned.

Then, as Russell and I turned to look at each other, our eyes filled with tears.

CHAPTER 6

A Wrenching Surrender

One does not surrender a life in an instant.
That which is lifelong can only be surrendered in a lifetime.
— Elisabeth Elliot

The morning was filled with pre-op tests. We were then informed that Russell would be admitted to surgery as soon as the operating theater was available.

While your loved one is the most special person in the world to *you*, a hospital's busyness makes you painfully aware that he's just the next guy in the assembly line that day... thank God for hospitals, nevertheless.

The Pre-Op

By 11:30 a.m., Russ was in the pre-op area, resting in a narrow bed on wheels. The room was configured like a horseshoe, with patients in their individual cots separated by curtains on both sides.

Russell was wrapped in a plastic blanket puffed up with warm air. He looked like a giant caterpillar, with a floppy blue shower cap on his head and purple socks on his feet. The room was freezing, but at least Russell was warm and comfortable.

Russell smiled bravely at me. We reassured each other that God was watching over us and we'd soon hear good news. We both desperately wanted to believe that.

Release and Surrender

At noon, the surgeon arrived. He explained how the flow of the afternoon would go, and handed me a pager that was to go off when the surgery was finished. That would be my signal to call him. Then, he surprised us both by reaching out for our hands.

"Let's pray," he said.

Gratefully, we bowed our heads. Russell and I both marveled at the many touches of God's grace we'd already experienced that morning.

He said a quick prayer and the time was up. It was a wrenching moment of surrender. I now had to release Russell to strangers—experts, certainly, but strangers nonetheless. I could no longer protect him—or so I felt.

I cried out in my spirit for God to look after him. Then, there was barely time for a quick kiss before he was whisked across the floor and out of the room through large swinging double doors. My heart went after him.

CHAPTER 7

A Touch of the Absurd

We sail within a vast sphere, ever drifting in uncertainty,
driven from end to end.
— Blaise Pascal

W hen I returned to the waiting area, Carmen had already left. Now Craig, a good friend of Russell's, was sitting with Janet.

We all headed to the cafeteria for lunch. I was consumed with my own thoughts, and only half heard the animated conversation of these two raconteurs.

An Unexpected Twist

Only a short time had gone by when I suddenly spotted Russell's surgeon across the room talking with another man.

"I must be seeing things," I said to my friends. "That looks like Russell's surgeon."

"We've only been here 20 minutes!" exclaimed Janet. "Are you sure?"

"It certainly looks like him," I said, incredulous. "I guess there's only one way to find out."

As I began making my way through the crowded tables, the doctor caught my eye. He signaled that he wanted to finish the conversation he was having with his colleague.

"I'll come over to your table and talk to you in just a second," he indicated.

"It's him," I reported as I returned to my friends. "And he's coming to join us."

We were all baffled. I also noticed that I was shaking.

Mixed Emotions

The doctor finally came and sat down.

"We removed the tumor," he announced, "It was very quick."

"Evidently," I said, with an edge of sarcasm. "Did *you* do the actual surgery, or was it someone else?" I had visions of Russell lying in the operating theatre at the hands of a junior assistant, while this man ordered sushi for lunch.

"Oh, no, I did the surgery," he said with flushing cheeks. "I paged you and also called your cell phone, but you didn't pick up."

I quickly looked down at the pager and saw that, in fact, it *had* gone off.

"I'm terribly sorry," I said, chagrined. "You'd said it would take about an hour… I didn't look at it or hear my cell phone."

"No problem," he said affably. "So, we caught the tumor early; we got it all and things look good."

"Oh, thank God!" We all broke into laughter and applause.

"I have some images here if you want to see them," he said as he pulled out some 8" x 10" photocopies. "Is it okay if I show you in front of your friends?"

A Touch of the Absurd

I momentarily froze. The request seemed absolutely bizarre and very indiscreet. His sudden presence in the cafeteria was surreal enough, but now he was proposing to show my husband's intimate body parts to strangers at the lunch table. Despite my inner struggle, I trusted Janet and Craig and knew they wouldn't mind. So desperate to know everything, I found myself nodding in approval.

The pictures were close-ups of the 1.5 x 2.2 centimeters bloody blob and surrounding tissue. Everything looked horribly raw and inflamed.

I felt sick and squeamish, but listened attentively. He said other potential surgeries might be needed down the road—including removing the prostate gland. He spoke as though Russell's body was like a car with parts that could be torn out or replaced, as needed.

"You're talking about Jack LaLanne, y'know," Craig blurted suddenly. He *also* was bothered by the surgeon's detached report about his dear friend.

"Excuse me?" asked the doctor.

"Russell is like Jack LaLanne," explained Craig. "He's a body builder. He takes really good care of himself—he's not your average guy."

"Uh, okay," said the doctor, not tracking where this was going.

"I wouldn't be so sure he'll need all those surgeries," said Craig with a wry smile.

"Bless you, Craig," I exhaled.

By now, my head was throbbing and I was quite nauseous. I could barely stay at the table, much less entertain any thought of future surgeries.

The only thing I chose to focus on was that the cancer had been caught early, the tumor was successfully removed, and Russell would be going home that same afternoon. It was selective listening, but it was all my frightened heart was able to handle at the time.

CHAPTER 8
TROUBLING SIGNS

Intuition is a spiritual faculty and does not explain, but simply
points the way.
— Florence Scovel Shinn

Arriving home from the hospital, Russell and I felt indescribable relief and joy. How bad could things really be, if he'd had surgery in the morning but was allowed home that same afternoon?

We thanked God for letting us catch the tumor early. We thanked Him for the care, the friends, the grace, the good report. We thanked Him for life.

We thought it was over.

Post-op Developments

Part of Russell's post-op care included wearing a catheter for a week. Though he felt well overall, by the third day the catheter began to hurt.

I phoned the doctor. He said it was normal.

Then, Russ also started bleeding.

I phoned the doctor again. He said it was normal.

Then, the pain and the bleeding increased.

I phoned the doctor again. This time, he sounded surprised and unsure. Maybe it wasn't normal, he said. I became afraid and suspicious.

"If the bleeding does not stop," the doctor said, "we'll have to go in again to cauterize the wound."

"You mean, do surgery again *on the same wound?*" I asked, shocked. "Didn't you cauterize it the first time?"

His answered in circles… he was vague… he let slip he had not done many of these procedures.

Suddenly, all the events of the past few days collided in my brain: the speedy surgery, the doctor's presence in the cafeteria, sharing private photos at the lunch table, the roundabout answers…

"I don't trust him anymore," I told Russell. "I think we need to get a second opinion."

"So do I," he agreed lying in considerable pain. "Something's not right."

CHAPTER 9

MORE BAD NEWS

Hope deferred makes the heart sick.
— Proverbs 13:12

We navigated the rest of a difficult week for Russ. Finally, Monday came and the catheter was removed.

Russell felt instant relief. He told the doctor how much it had hurt. The doctor seemed unaware that wearing it for seven days could become so painful. We both found that unsettling, but were even more unprepared for what happened next.

Without preamble, our specialist informed us that though he'd successfully removed the tumor during surgery, he'd also taken tissue samples of Russell's bladder wall and sent these to the lab for testing. This seemed appropriate and we followed his reasoning... until he stated flatly: "The tissues tested positive for high-grade cancer."

I gasped.

"The good news is that so far, the cancer is non-invasive and has not penetrated muscle wall—at least in the area that I took the tissue from. The bad news is, if it has penetrated into the muscle wall somewhere else, or is close to invading the muscle wall, we have to take the bladder out."

Russell's face paled. I gripped my stomach.

The doctor then drew a quick diagram illustrating the three layers of the bladder wall. As long as the cancer stayed within the inner layer (the *transitional epithelium*, he explained), the cancer was contained.

But if it had spread into the nearby *lamina propria*, or even deeper into the muscle layer, it could then break through and quickly spread to other parts of the body.

This cancer wanted to kill.

"Fortunately, when I nipped your bladder to take the tissue samples, I didn't perforate the muscle wall," he admitted.

We found that a frightening confession.

"But, we do need to take more samples next week," he announced bluntly.

"Next week?" protested Russell. "But I'm still bleeding from the surgery! And my prostate is bruised!"

"Your prostrate is not bruised," countered our doctor defensively. "And there's no time to waste."

We sensed some fear in him, that perhaps he had not done a careful-enough job the first time. Something felt terribly wrong.

"We need to think about it," Russell told him.

Thanking him, we walked out the door.

We never went back.

CHAPTER 10

AN EAGLE IN SCRUBS

Hope begins in the dark, the stubborn hope that if you just show up
and try to do the right thing, the dawn will come.
You wait and watch and work. You don't give up.
— Anne LaMott

By now, we'd put the word out to our community of friends: We were looking for a second opinion.

Within just a few days, we had a referral to one of the best bladder specialists in the country. Providentially, he worked not far away, at the University of Southern California's Norris Cancer Center, a renowned facility. The doctor's schedule was booked solid, but thankfully, his staff managed to squeeze us in.

In less than two weeks, we were in his office.

Russell had continued with intermittent bleeding and pain during this time, so we were keen to come under the care of someone we trusted.

The new doctor met us in between surgeries. He came into the exam room wearing scrubs and an American flag for a bandana. Middle-aged, slim, with piercing sky-blue eyes, he reminded me of an eagle. His energy was calm and steady.

Russell explained his journey up to this point. The surgeon listened attentively, then asked: "Has anyone taken a look at you since the surgery?"

Russell shook his head. "Let's see what's going on in there," the surgeon said.

Russ lay on the exam table with a monitor overhead. By now, we knew the drill.

Using the urinary catheter, the surgeon traveled it up inside till he reached Russell's bladder. This time, the sight was shocking:

The tissues that had once been smooth and pink now looked angry and swollen; the bladder was puffy and disfigured, especially where the tumor had been. There also were white skin fragments floating around like ghostly butter-flies. Clearly, the surgery had been executed roughly.

"Your prostate looks bruised!" the doctor exclaimed.

"Tell me about it!" said Russell. "That's what I told our other surgeon, but he denied it. As if I didn't know what I was feeling!"

My heart was pounding. I turned to Russell and said: "I know we haven't discussed this privately, but we're switching doctors right this minute."

Russell said, "I totally agree!"

The surgeon nodded. "That's what I would do."

Finding this doctor's professional manner so reassuring, we immediately began to ask about possible treatments.

Sensing Russell and I were anxious to push through this hurdle and get on with our lives, the doctor advised us gently: "You need to have a healthy respect for this cancer."

His comment came as a jolt.

He continued: "This is the worst kind of cancer. It will not even respond to chemo."

We both froze.

"Then what options do we have?" Russell finally asked.

"If you're a candidate, we might try treatments of BCG," the doctor said thoughtfully. "It's Bacillus Calmette-Guerin, a type of bacterium used in tuberculosis vaccines; It stimulates the bladder's own immune system so that it fights any toxins in the bladder itself—in this case, the cancer."

"How will we know if he's a candidate?" I asked.

"I first need to see his lab reports and the CT scans from his surgery," the doctor explained. "That will tell me a lot."

"I'll get those and bring them to you as fast as I can," I told him.

Russ said: "Our other doctor said he saw nothing in the CT scan, yet the tumor was obviously there."

"That's why I want to take a look," explained our new specialist. "Then, we need to go in and do a biopsy."

"Right away?" Russell asked, worried.

"No, you need time to heal," he said. "This is June… let's plan on three months from now, in mid-September."

While we agreed that another operation right away made no sense, we also felt uneasy about waiting three months. *What if the cancer punched through the muscle wall before then?*

Unfortunately, our time was up. The doctor was due in surgery, so this question would have to wait till another appointment.

And so began a new climb up our Everest, taking a different path this time. It would still prove to be tougher and more terrifying than we ever expected. But this time, at least, we felt we were in better hands.

CHAPTER 11
WORSE THAN EXPECTED

The first step to victory is to understand the enemy.
— Corrie Ten Boom

I spent the next couple of days collecting Russell's lab reports and CT scans from the first hospital.

As I was dropping them off at USC Norris, I ran into our new specialist, again in between surgeries. He was sitting at his desk in a small, unassuming office eating a salad. He invited me to sit.

I was bursting with questions.

"If the cancer is in the first two tissue layers but wants to penetrate the bladder wall, shouldn't we do the surgery sooner?" I asked him anxiously.

"Unfortunately, my schedule is booked solid for the next several weeks, and then I'll be out of the country on vacation," he answered.

"But what if you get a cancellation?" I pressed. "That must happen."

"We do need to wait," he explained. "I can't get an accurate reading until he's healed."

"I see... but isn't it dangerous to wait?" I persisted.

Sensing my anxiety, he paused and said: "It *is* a calculated risk. But this cancer most likely began years ago. Was your husband exposed to second-hand smoke or industrial equipment?"

"His father was a chain smoker," I explained. "And he's been around smokers from years of his work in the theater."

The surgeon nodded.

"What are our chances of success with the BCG vaccines?" I asked.

"About 25 to 30 percent."

I looked aghast.

Observing my fear, he said: "I know you want specifics and guarantees. But you're just going to have to trust me."

"What about natural therapies and nutrition?" I pressed, looking for a ray of hope. "Do you approve of trying things like vitamin-C therapy and beta-glucan supplements?"

Waving his hand dismissively, he said: "It's fine if you want to try any of those. But this is a very aggressive cancer. There's a 95-percent chance he's going to have to have his bladder out... if not now, sometime down the line."

"You mean to save his life?"

"Yes," he nodded.

I thanked him for his time, left him the reports, and walked back to my car, shaking from head to toe.

CHAPTER 12

HEAVINGS OF THE SOUL

Being deeply loved by someone gives you strength,
while loving someone deeply gives you courage.
— Lao Tzu

The USC surgeon's prognosis was so devastating, I couldn't bring myself to tell Russell. I feared the news would dangerously demoralize him, weakening the hope and strength he was going to need to fight the battle ahead.

Count the Cost

What I hadn't considered, however, was how carrying this secret would affect me. The thought of losing Russell triggered a fear so deep, I could hardly breathe.

Only once before in my life had I experienced a comparable blow—the kind that makes your head throb and your legs stagger like a drunk's —and that was at the death of my mother.

Her sudden passing had been so devastating that throughout my life I experienced "happiness anxiety"—i.e., a deep dread that any real happiness might be suddenly ripped away from me at any time.

The Substance of Our Faith

"We don't know what our faith is truly made of until it is tested," a friend said to me.

How true. The Bible says all trials are tests to reveal where our trust really lies—whether on the Lord, ourselves, or on an endless list of other false gods such as talent, money, power, education, etc. Or in our case, perhaps doctors, treatments and medicines?

> **Beloved, do not be surprised at the painful trial you are suffering,
> as though something strange were happening to you.**
> **— 1 Peter 4:12**

This prognosis drove me to God with a desperation like that of the Shunammite woman in the Old Testament (2 Kings 4:18-38). After the death of her only son—the treasure of her heart—she clung to the Prophet Elisha's feet in the deepest distress.

And God, working His power through Elisha, brought the boy back to life and restored him to his grateful mother.

I, too, clung to God's feet in my prayer times, asking for this same deliverance for my husband.

No Fingertip Prayers

> It is the burning lava of the soul
> that has a furnace within
> —a very volcano of grief and sorrow—
> it is that burning lava of prayer
> that finds its way to God.
> No prayer ever reaches God's heart
> which does not come from our hearts.
> — Charles Spurgeon

If you've ever been in a desperate situation, you know that is *not* the time for polite prayers. Fasting and fervent intercession, giant heavings of the soul day and night—those are what is needed to fight such a battle.

If our Savior prayed this way, are we to do any less?

And so I fasted, studied the Scriptures, prayed in the mornings with Russell, and also throughout the day. I memorized verses, and wrote in my journal. Sometimes, I awoke in the middle of the night and prayed till dawn. I shed many, many tears.

> **During the days of Jesus' life on earth, He offered up prayers and petitions
> with loud cries and tears to the One Who could save Him from death,
> and He was heard because of His reverent submission.**
> **— Hebrews 5:7**

Wrestling with Fear

Fear also gripped my heart. Was God going to heal Russell? Was that part of the plan? I didn't dare hope for deliverance if it wasn't meant to be.

In addition to the doctor's prognosis, I was tormented by the words that author Elisabeth Elliot spoke at a lecture I'd once attended.

"Be careful what you fear," she warned.

I never forgot those words, and they haunted me now. The same thought is articulated in Job 3:35: "What I feared has come upon me, what I dreaded has happened to me."

Fear comes from the enemy of our souls, and he delights to torture us with it. Was my fear of losing Russell going to be a self-fulfilling prophecy? Had my fear attracted his illness in some way? Would my unresolved issues impede his healing?

A drowning man cannot throw himself a rope. I had to get some help.

CHAPTER 13
TAKING PERSONAL INVENTORY

You cannot help but learn more as you take the world into your hands.
Take it up reverently, for it is an old piece of clay,
with millions of thumbprints on it.
— John Updike

Russell was meeting with a friend and pastor named Murray (not his real name) to work through his own fears. To Russell, this cancer somehow felt like a test—one he might fail.

The men invited me to participate with them in these counseling sessions, and I found Murray's discernment, compassion and skill simply breathtaking. He had a gift for uncovering the root causes of an issue, then helping one bring these broken and unsanctified places under the healing touch of Christ.

In one session, Murray asked Russ if there had been any curses spoken over him during his life. Russell suddenly got very emotional.

"I remember cursing myself about two years ago," he confessed. "I was feeling particularly exhausted and worn out from work and wished I could just die. Seconds after doing it, I felt a chill and thought: *Uh-oh, you just opened a door.*"

Murray expertly guided Russell through repenting of those ill words and feelings, receiving forgiveness, and renewing his mind with the truths of Scripture.

Murray also prayed to God to free Russell from any residual demonic oppression, and for God to strengthen him in the inner man.

> **I have always noted that Satan prefers to attack us when we are in a low and weak state, rather than at any other time.**
> **— Charles Spurgeon**

Witnessing how he helped heal and fortify Russ, I asked Murray to work with me, too. Russell understood I was afraid—though he had no idea how much—and he completely supported my need, never questioning my request for private sessions.

My Own Inner Healing Journey

I shared with Murray the dim statistics about the BCG treatments—stats that were not only frightening in and of themselves, but that also triggered a flood of fear from my own past.

> **O my Father, my God, help me to wrestle with this temptation, and make me more than a conqueror through Your dear Son.**
> **— Charles Spurgeon**

Under Murray's expert care, I experienced a deep inner healing of early wounds stemming from my mother's fatal accident. Through the guidance of the Holy Spirit, many unresolved thoughts and feelings surfaced. Some were primal and terrifying, having to do with the moment of death when the soul separates from the body.

Though spiritually inclined, my mother was not a Christian before she died. However, I cannot know what may have transpired between her and God during those final tragic minutes when the private jet lost power and went into a nosedive.

To make matters worse, my mother had been terrified of flying her entire life.

> **The purposes of a man's heart are like deep waters, but a man of understanding draws them out.**
> **— Proverbs 20:5**

Murray helped expose all these jumbled issues, and aided me in renouncing the distorted thinking that I nurtured after this childhood trauma. His healing prayers were also a balm to my soul. We took everything to the cross, to the finished work of Christ, and "put on" a more-biblical perspective to replace the lies. It was *so* cleansing and liberating!

Some of my wounds had also allowed demonic strongholds in my heart. Powerful warfare prayers also became an integral part of my healing process.

Lastly, we also tackled whether my fear of loss might have "attracted" Russell's cancer in some way, or could even compromise his recovery. As I experienced inner healing from these early wounds,

> You were taught... to put off your old self, which is being corrupted by its deceitful desires; to be made new in the attitude of your minds; and to put on the new self...
> — Ephesians 4:22-24a

this fear no longer found a foothold... and simply vanished.

By the end of my sessions I was a new person—spiritually, mentally and emotionally. Thank God for Murray, thank God for the Holy Spirit, thank God for the Truth... it set me free!

The Ongoing Heartache

Despite these huge breakthroughs, a burning question still lingered: *Was it God's will to heal Russell?*

Though I pored over Scriptures and pressed in during prayer, I could not discern an answer. And not knowing was torture.

I decided to seek the counsel of yet another gifted pastor, whom I deeply trusted and believed could help.

CHAPTER 14
DIVINE PARTNERSHIPS

Faith is being sure of what we hope for,
and certain of what we do not see.
— Hebrews 11:1

Jeff and Patsy Perry lead a vibrant church in Missouri called the St. Louis Family Church. They also direct an international relief ministry called Service International.

Over the last decade, their ministry's teams have helped hundreds of thousands of disaster victims in Oklahoma, Mississippi, Louisiana, Haiti, and the Philippines. Their reach *also* extends to the nation of Kosovo, where for years they've helped war-torn families rebuild their communities.

In addition, Jeff and Patsy direct a once-a-month ministry in Los Angeles called "Third Tuesday." It equips Christians who work in media and entertainment to stay true to their calling and touch the world for Christ through their respective creative endeavors.

Russell and I were regular attendees of these Third-Tuesday meetings. We considered them a privilege.

Pastor Jeff understood the world of show biz, with all its craziness, wonder and potential. His passionate exhortations to shine brightly for Christ and run with endurance the race marked out for us always strengthened our hearts and resolve.

Another special blessing of these meetings was connecting with other brothers and sisters who, like the Old Testament prophet Nehemiah, knew what it was to build with one hand and hold a sword in the other!

Oh God, Hear My Prayer

So it was that on a third Tuesday, I was driving myself to the monthly meeting. Russ was tied up that night at work and could not join me. I was in agony and beseeched God to please meet me there and show me the way. What was I to hope for? Was He going to heal Russell? What did the future hold?

I prayed inwardly through the whole evening. At the end of the event, I went down to the front of the room. Pastor Jeff had begun to pray with someone, so I poured out my heart to Patsy, a woman of deep strength and discernment. She is *also* a furnace of faith!

Patsy immediately understood my pain and began ministering powerfully to my heart.

Faith Comes by Hearing

She encouraged me to trust God and believe in His willingness to heal. She shared stories of cancer healings in California, Texas, and in their own church in St. Louis. She suggested books and resources.

Her conviction that God *does* heal, is *willing* to heal, and *wanted* to heal *Russell* was so absolute, I found my own faith for healing sputter to life for the very first time. I could actually *feel* the Holy Spirit speaking through her... and I began to *believe!*

Divine Instructions

When Pastor Jeff became available, Patsy and I explained the situation and he began to pray for me. This pastor is a mighty man of God, and I will never forget his prayer. The Holy Spirit was powerfully present, and I paid rapt attention to every word.

Jeff began by praising God for His compassion, power and mercy, and his tone was serious. He then asked God to give Russell and me wisdom, endurance, and *strategy* to know how to best fight this battle.

In recounting it here, it sounds so simple. But suddenly, with that one word—*strategy*—I experienced a thunderbolt of understanding. This was a concept close to my core. As a prayer intercessor (those who stand in the gap for others in prayer), I recognized that this was a military term; a call to stealth in combat for those at war with a ruthless and cruel enemy.

Jeff kept praying, and God started downloading the entire blueprint into my spirit: There wouldn't be *one* divine stroke of instant healing for Russell, but rather a series of strategic milestones that would unfold step by step as we moved forward *in faith*. We *could* win this war... but it would be one battle at a time.

I "saw" in my spirit that the fight would be hard... harder than I had ever imagined. It would also be dangerous because we could fail. Victory would require a level of discipline, courage and grit that was unprecedented. Unwavering faith and focus would be essential.

I physically felt the heaviness of the assignment fall on me. But the prospect of victory also made my heart swell. It was a defining moment. The warrior in me stepped up, put on her full armor and declared herself ready to battle.

The stakes were life and death. The enemy was formidable. But victory was possible. Those were my instructions.

This all transpired in a matter of minutes. When I opened my eyes, I was no longer the same person. I'd arrived a jellyfish, but was leaving a warrior armed with vision and resolve. All my fear and doubts had vanished, and I *believed* with every fiber of my being that God *would* heal Russell.

Though we would still have to walk through the fire, our *strategies* would now be fueled with the weapons of an unshakable faith and determination.

Anything less and we'd career off the cliff.

From Despair to Breakthrough

I don't think either Pastor Jeff or Patsy knew the enormity of the breakthrough they had facilitated that night. The Holy Spirit was moving so deeply in my spirit, I could hardly talk. But I did my best to thank them profusely, then left.

The first battle had already been won—in my heart!

> **The prayer offered in faith will make the sick person well;**
> **the Lord will raise him up.**
> **— James 5:15**

CHAPTER 15
A HOLY MOMENT

Some trust in chariots, and some in horses,
but we trust in the name of the Lord our God.
— Psalm 20:7

Armed with a vision for healing and a heart burning with resolve, I arrived home to Russell. I shared with him my newfound faith that God *was* willing to heal him, and that we *could* be victorious over this cancer.

The Holy Spirit fell in a powerful way, and stirred deeply in Russell's heart. As my husband listened and saw my confidence, his faith also was kindled. I saw Russell's fears vanish and his spirit lift... and he *believed!*

Linking Hearts

That very instant, a holy moment took place. Our hearts linked up with divine determination for the healing journey ahead—a journey we would take together step by step, unwavering, no matter what lay ahead, and with our eyes fixed on Jesus, the "Author and Perfecter of our faith" (Hebrews 12:2).

CHAPTER 16

TESTS OF FAITH

Where there is no counsel, the people fall,
but in the multitude of counselors there is safety.
— Proverbs 11:14

E very vision from God will be tested and our test came quickly. We were
waiting with bated breath to hear what our USC Norris surgeon would
say about Russell's CT scans.

Whereas our first urologist had said the technician's report did not reveal
any growths, our Norris surgeon said the scan clearly showed the original tumor.
The difference was: The first doctor just *read a report prepared by a technician*,
whereas the Norris specialist *examined the scan himself*.

This taught us the importance of one's actual doctor examining these types of
scans, not just the behind-the-scenes technicians who have considerably inferior
training and expertise.

Mixed News

We were then hugely encouraged when our Norris surgeon then said that the more
recent scans looked clear with no other detectable growths or abnormalities.

Thank you, God! Big exhale!

However, he warned, the cancer was definitely there, growing in the tissues
at the molecular level.

This warning sent shudders up our spines.

If Russell were to need his bladder removed to prevent the spread of cancer
(this is called a *cystectomy*), it would mean he'd have to live out his days with a
tube protruding from his abdominal wall. This is called a *urostomy*.

From an opening called a *stoma*, this tube would drain his fluid waste into a pouch strapped to a flat surface somewhere on his body. The bag would need to be monitored and emptied regularly.

If it meant saving his life, we agreed that we would not hesitate to take this step. But if we could keep Russell whole, this vigorous Renaissance man could continue living an active and productive life for many years to come.

The Tug of War

Hope and fear... progress and setbacks. Our hearts were in a tug-of-war.

The surgeon reiterated that before Russell had his next biopsy, we should wait three months (until September) for him to heal. This exam would reveal how infected his bladder had become, and in what layers the malignancy was lurking.

Fighting Back

For us, three months was an agonizing eternity. Weren't we just giving the cancer a free pass, allowing it to keep spreading and birthing toxic cells that might perforate the bladder wall and attack the rest of the body?

I was struggling with the timeline. However, Russell trusted the doctor's request to wait until he was healed, so they could get an accurate reading.

And so, it was decided that the BCG treatment would be put on hold for three months.

But that didn't mean we could not assertively move forward in alternative—and *strategic*—ways.

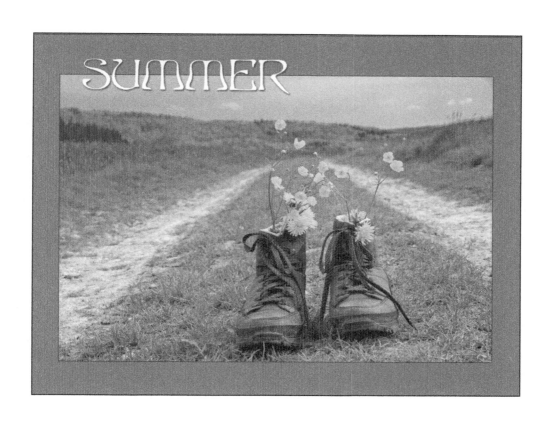

CHAPTER 17

A STRATEGIC MINDSET

If you would successfully wrestle with Satan,
make the Holy Scriptures your daily commune.
Out of this sacred Word
continually draw your armor and ammunition.
— Charles Spurgeon

Research shows that the kind of people who survive natural disasters, assaults, crises and/or illnesses are those who fight back, determined to overcome the adversity. Depression, doubt, fear, hopelessness, despair—these are the enemies of survival and healing.[1]

Our Three-Month Strategy

While we waited for September's biopsy, we chose to engage in a rigorous regimen that included spiritual, nutritional and physical disciplines. We were motivated by faith that these would not only help Russell fight the cancer, but might even defeat the malignancy completely.

We gave ourselves three months. Our hope was, when September arrived and our Norris urologist did the biopsy, we'd hear three magical words: "He's completely healed."

So we repeatedly meditated on the following holy words and their meanings, both clear-cut *and* implied:

---

1   Siebert, A. (1996). *The Survivor Personality: Why Some People Are Stronger, Smarter, and More Skillful at Handling Life's Difficulties... and How You Can Be, Too.* New York: Berkeley Publishing Group.

> **My word that goes out from my mouth, it will not return to me empty,
> but will accomplish what I desire and achieve the purpose for which I sent it.
> — Isaiah 55:11**

And out of this meditation came the following disciplines or regimens for every possible aspect of our lives.

SPIRITUAL STRATEGIES

I. Personal Strategies

- We began our mornings in quality time with the Lord, poring over the Scriptures (see the verse listings on page 95).
- We also kept a spiritual journal, which included writing those Scriptural promises we felt God was giving us. These literally jumped off the pages and into our hearts. We also chronicled our feelings, doubts, hopes, and promptings of the Spirit.
- We memorized key Scriptures, turned them into prayers, then prayed these back to the Lord. We did this together and individually.
- We prayed these Scriptures inwardly, throughout each day as we went about our business.
- If God woke us up in the middle of the night, we willingly got up to pray... and to listen, as He often had direction for our hearts.
- I fasted and prayed as God directed, for short and long stretches at a time. (We did not feel it was healthy for Russell to fast.)

I cannot stress enough how life-changing these strategies proved to be. While God always wants us to have a consistent prayer life (so we can always be in close communication with Him), this is more critical than ever when one is going through a dangerous trial and depending on God's moment-by-moment wisdom to make the right choices.

Truth for the Journey

As we drew close to Him, these truths seeped into the marrow of our bones:

1. God never lies, therefore His Word is true.

2. If His Word is true, then I can believe His promises.

3. If I can believe His promises, then no matter what the circumstances *look like* in the natural realm, they eventually have to *line up in obedience to God's will.*

4. Until things *do* line up, I can continue to cling to His Word. In this way, I can defeat the waves of doubt and fear when they come, and experience the "peace that surpasses understanding" (Philippians 4:7).

This is the substance of our *faith*!

> **You who call on the Lord, give yourselves no rest**
> **and give Him no rest.**
> **— Isaiah 62:6-7**

II. Group Prayer

In addition to our personal disciplines, we also organized several in-person and "virtual" sessions of intercessory prayer with friends from all over the country—and even other parts of the world (see details in Chapter 19.)

III. Prayer from Church Leaders

We shared our trial with our church leaders. They were supportive and compassionate. They also anointed Russell with oil and prayed over both of us.

IV. Seminars

The Lord led us to cross paths with an old friend whom we had not seen for years; today he has an international healing ministry. We quickly recognized this as a divine appointment, and his teaching offered tremendous emotional and spiritual equipping (see Chapter 18 for details).

NUTRITIONAL STRATEGIES

We'd always followed a healthy diet, but the cancer forced us to search deeper and learn about healing foods and regimens with proven track records. These approaches felt right and gave us a lot of strength. We followed them rigorously (see details in Chapter 20).

EXERCISE STRATEGIES

Regular exercise had always been a part of our lives, but we now took special care with our routines. Interval training (high-to-low-intensity exercises) and weight training were a positive outlet for stress, kept us strong, and helped eliminate toxins—a hugely important aspect to healing.

CHAPTER 18

Overcoming the Enemy

Joshua fought the Amalekites as Moses had ordered,

and Moses, Aaron and Hur went to the top of the hill.

As long as Moses held up his hands, the Israelites were winning,

but whenever he lowered his hands, the Amalekites were winning.

When Moses' hands grew tired, they took a stone and put it under him

and he sat on it. Aaron and Hur held his hands up—one on one side,

one on the other—so that his hands remained steady till sunset.

So Joshua overcame the Amalekite army with the sword.

— Exodus 17:10-13

Spiritual Resources for Spiritual Battles

Scripture repeatedly reminds us that we cannot win spiritual battles relying on our human strength; we need spiritual resources to succeed at spiritual assignments.

In Exodus 17, we read that Israel was engaged in a great battle with its enemies.

Moses, standing on top of a hill, discovered that while he held up his arms, the armies of Israel were winning the battle in the valley below.

But it was a prolonged battle, and to keep his arms steady from sunrise to sunset, he needed the support of two friends on either side of him to help hold up his arms.

> Prayer is not preparation for work, it is the work. Prayer is not preparation for the battle, it is the battle.
> — Oswald Chambers

The *strategy* worked and Israel won the battle. Again, the operative word here is *strategy.*

Know Your Enemy

In John 10:10, Jesus warns his disciples, "The thief comes only to steal, kill and destroy." In light of this teaching, it was clear to us that the spiritual origins of this cancer came straight from the pit of hell.

Thankfully, the Bible has *lots* to say about how to face our archenemy and overcome. Therefore, we knew a *spiritual strategy* would be an essential component in winning the battle for Russell's health.

That meant not just leaning on God for wisdom, direction and strength, but also equipping our army of prayer partners everywhere with greater focus.

A Global Army of Prayer Warriors

By mid-summer, our prayer network had grown to about 100 people, and spread as far as Mexico and India! We let everyone know we were working with a three-month window for Russell's healing.

I never shared the doctor's dark prognosis, since I had not yet told Russell and also did not wish to dampen anyone else's faith, either. But I did inform them that the cancer was "so malignant it would not respond to chemotherapy."

We also shared that our goal was to arrive at the surgery in September and hear the surgeon say: "He's completely healed."

A Strengthening of the Heart

As we shared our vision, God moved in people's hearts. Friends everywhere declared themselves willing to partner with us and align with our God-given vision for healing.

Their declarations of love and support deeply touched our hearts. When people are there for you in your hour of deepest need, what can you say? "Thank you" is simply not enough. Without question, during this darkest of times, this outpouring of love and support was the most precious of blessings.

The Bad Days

Some days were really hard, especially when we were tired. We'd feel the enemy messing with our heads, ridiculing our efforts, hissing in our ear that death was just around the corner. Those days were horrific, but I'd be lying if I said we didn't have them.

> **Indeed, in our hearts we felt the sentence of death. But, this happened that we might not rely on ourselves but on God, Who raises from the dead.**
> **— 2 Corinthians 1:9**

Embracing Life Ministries

Jonathan Hunter was an old friend of Russell's, but several years had passed since they had connected. One day we "coincidentally" ran into Jonathan at a restaurant. In catching up, we found out about his ministry, "Embracing Life." It provides tools, encouragement and strength to people with life-altering conditions—including cancer. (See details under List of Resources, page 95.)

Sad to say, we knew of several people who were struggling with serious health issues of their own. So, we spontaneously organized a special Embracing Life Seminar for these friends and ourselves, plus a few others who Jonathan also knew.

> **The darkness retreats in the face of someone who knows who he is in Christ.**
> **— Jonathan Hunter**

The teaching was deep and full of wisdom. It increased our discernment about how to recognize the enemy's tactics, heal unresolved areas of weakness and mentally prepare—for the long haul. This proved to be especially helpful as, unbeknownst to us, there were tough times and hard setbacks still ahead.

Jonathan's book, *More Life! Breaking Free... from the Spirit of Death*, also led us to new understanding of the spiritual devilry unleashed on the minds and bodies of Christians with vulnerable conditions. It gave us Scriptural tools and equipping about our authority in Christ when we experienced the enemy's slings and arrows aimed at destroying our faith and vision for healing.

Remember Others

When we stepped back and took stock, we marveled at God's lavish provision of so many resources to help us be more than conquerors through Him Who loved us. He, also, always delivered each one at the perfect time.

In addition, we felt confident that our outgoing spiritual efforts—lifting up, praying for and encouraging others who were hurting—pleased the Lord. We are all called to care about the needs of others, not just our own needs. So we were faithful and consistent in prayer for them.

> All you who bend the bow, shoot against sin and Satan.
> Spare no arrows, for your enemies are rebels against God.
> Go up against them, put your feet upon their necks,
> fear not, neither be dismayed, for the battle is the Lord's,
> and the Lord will deliver your enemy into your hands.
> — Charles Spurgeon

CHAPTER 19

THE PRAYER STRATEGIES

You have the power over angels, who will fly at your will.

You will have the power over fire, and water,

and the elements of the earth. You have the power

to make your voice heard beyond the stars.

Where the thunders die out in silence, your voice

shall wake the echoes of eternity. The ear of God

shall listen, and the hand of God shall yield to your will.

God bids you cry "Thy will be done," and your will shall be done.

When you can plead His promise, then your will is His will.

— Charles Spurgeon

As we followed God's lead, our group-prayer times took on many shapes and sizes.

NOTE: I've listed several types of intercession below, but if you or your loved one are fighting a serious battle, you can shape your prayer sessions in any way you feel led. What I share here is by no means a formula of any kind, but simply how God led us in our particular situation.

Overview of Prayer Sessions

We organized prayer sessions in our Los Angeles home for those who lived in the area. Our group sizes ranged from five to 30 people, and sessions lasted anywhere from two to four hours, depending on the event.

> **Call upon me in the day of trouble; I will deliver you, and you will honor me.**
> **— Psalm 50:15**

Preparing Hearts

We always began our prayer times with praise and worship. Fortunately, we had many friends who were musicians and happy to bless us with their gifting. When they were not available, we played a selection of worship music from CDs.

Praise helps us move into the spirit realm and open hearts to God's greatness. Even though we may be weighed down with many anxieties and sorrows, our soul wants to soar in the heavenly realms—that is its home! And once you begin praising, it's as if the angels themselves stoop down to lift you up.

Hard though it is, it's always good to get our eyes off ourselves and onto the magnificence and all-sufficiency of our God. Regardless of our pressing circumstances, we can all remember a long list of wondrous things God has done in the past that we can praise Him for—starting with our salvation and the very glorious person of Christ himself.

Kites of Praise

As we allowed our prayers and songs of thanksgiving to waft upwards, they became like multicolored kites, riding on the breezes of our praise and reaching heavenward to our Father, Who delights in releasing comfort, power and blessing in return.

> **Shout for joy to the LORD,**
> **all the earth,**
> **worship the LORD with gladness;**
> **come before Him with joyful songs.**
> **Know that the LORD is God.**
> **It is He Who made us,**
> **and we are His; we are His people,**
> **the sheep of His pasture.**
> **— Psalm 100:1-3**

Crafted Prayer

On one Sunday afternoon, a group of 10 of us got together for a time of what author Graham Cooke calls "crafted prayer."[2]

---

2   Cooke, G. (2004). *Crafted Prayer*. Grand Rapids: Chosen Books.

After a sweet time of praise and worship, we asked people to spend several quiet minutes in prayer alone with God, before we prayed together as a group.

We gave them pads of paper and asked them to write down any Scripture verses or promptings by the Holy Spirit—if any—about Russell's battle with cancer.

The principle here is to not only pray in the will of God, but to pray back to Him the very things He was telling us He wants to do!

> **To see your prayers answered, enter God's presence with thanksgiving and worship.**
> **Then, rest in your secret place and meditate on His Scripture and words to you.**
> **Ask the Lord: "What do You want to do in these circumstances?"**
> **Then, listen and wait until the Lord answers and directs you how to pray.**
> **— Graham Cooke**

You can take as much time as you want with this contemplative session before the Lord. Graham Cooke practices an hour, two hours, or even up to half a day of contemplation.

When the focus is specifically on healing prayer, Graham will also schedule ongoing prayer sessions, over a period of several weeks with the same people, until the breakthrough comes.

(For more-in-depth case studies of physical healing through the practice of sustained sessions of crafted prayer, please refer to Cooke's *Crafted Prayer*, which is listed in the Resources section at the end of this book.)

On that Sunday afternoon, our group only had a moderate window of time, so we asked that everyone sit silently before the Lord for about 20 minutes.

People found separate corners of the living room and prayed silently. Nobody spoke to each other or compared notes.

> **Prayer means not only talking to Him, but waiting before Him**
> **till the dust settles and the stream runs clear.**
> **— F.B. Meyer**

When we gathered back together, people began sharing their insights, Scripture verses and phrases. One after another we heard: *God wants to heal Russell.*

With each verse, our sense of excitement grew—cautiously.

Inwardly, we paused to consider if we were simply hearing people's wishful thinking: Was this simply our friends' desire to strengthen and encourage us, or was it truly the Holy Spirit?

But the same message was relayed, again and again in different words and Scripture verses, and all delivered with great conviction.

I reminded myself what God had revealed to me at the Third Tuesday gathering: God *could* and *would* heal Russell... so he and I decided to shake off our unbelief.

By the time everyone finished sharing, the sweetest spirit of peace had descended over us. We then entered into about half an hour of faith-filled group prayer. It was simply beautiful. After this, we parted ways, feeling a deep sense of joy and anticipation.

Fasting

The Bible refers to fasting as something that is good, profitable and powerful.

Jesus taught that fasting brings deliverance from demonic oppression (Matthew 17:21). Paul referred to fasting as a spiritual discipline, and a means of helping discern of God's will (Acts 13:2; 14:23). Fasting is also meant to help us focus completely on God and facilitate a breakthrough in our lives (Matthew 6:16-18).

I've had low blood pressure my whole life, so skipping meals for long stretches of time is not healthy for me. However, I did fast on those days when I did not have strenuous activities.

And I occasionally skipped a meal and prayed instead. I also abstained from several of my favorite foods throughout the summer and fall.

Group Intercession with Praise and Worship

> God is pleased to answer individual prayers,
> but at times He seems to say:
> "You may entreat my favor, but I will not see your face
> unless your brethren are with you."
> — Charles Spurgeon

For one of our sessions, we invited a large group of friends to join us for a time of praise and intercession. God had impressed upon Russell and I to use praise and worship as a strategic weapon against the enemy. Our example in Scripture was found in the Old Testament: 2 Chronicles 20:21-22.

In order to include those who could not attend our prayer time in person, we arranged for an 800 number that people could use from anywhere in the country.

Russell hooked up a microphone in our media room, where we held the meeting. This enabled those who called in to hear us, and we could hear them in turn, except for those who whispered their prayers! But, we know God heard them! In total, about 30 people participated.

In a stunning display of loyalty, East-Coast friends from Pittsburgh and Virginia called in, as well as people from all over California. Friends of all ages were represented, from a 15-year-old (who texted his friend's prayer requests throughout the afternoon!) up to those in their 70s.

> We do not want fingertip prayers that barely touch the burden. We need shoulder prayers that bear a load of earnestness and are not to be denied their desire.
> — Charles Spurgeon

One hour melted into two, then three, then four. As some people left, others arrived…a relay of athletes of the heart and spirit.

The Power of the Holy Spirit

The afternoon was filled with passionate prayer, quoting of Scripture and spontaneous songs of praise.

One friend laid hands on Russell and declared God's marvelous promises about healing and deliverance. Another anointed him with oil. There were also many outbursts of heartfelt joy, laughter and singing.

Our media room became holy ground, a sacred space. Friends turned in to priests and prophets, and placed Russell at the feet of Jesus—like those men in Mark 2:3-5, who lowered their lame friend from the roof into the living room of a home where Christ was preaching.

As everyone took turns lifting up arms for the battle on this hill of faith, Russell and I both felt our heavy burden lift. The relief was tangible!

We shook the gates of heaven that afternoon! In an overwhelming display of love and devotion from our friends, we were blessed beyond words as waves and waves of prayers, songs and Scriptures washed over us. It was unforgettable and transcendent.

> **Is anyone among you sick? Let them call the elders of the church and pray over them and anoint them with oil in the name of the Lord.**
> **— James 5:14**

Partners at Church

In addition to our pastors' prayers, the prayer-ministry team from our church prayed with us, and a member of the convalescent ministry even paid us a home visit. We felt incredibly supported!

When we were invited to share our journey at one of our church's Saturday night services, about 300 people were present. And God graciously moved in the hearts of several members, who spontaneously committed to pray for Russell's recovery. We kept everyone updated as things progressed.

Partners in Other Churches

When Joel Osteen's mother, Dodie, was 48 years old, she was diagnosed with liver cancer and given two weeks to live. The hospital sent her home saying there was nothing more they could do.

But thanks to her indomitable faith, Dodie embarked on a series of rigorous spiritual practices that included standing on God's promises and prayer. Gradually, over a two-year period, without ever undergoing any medical treatments, Dodie was completely healed.

> You are the God
> who performs miracles;
> You display Your power
> among the peoples.
> — Psalm 77:14

Her little book, *Healed of Cancer*, chronicles this powerful testimony. When Russell and I read it, her story strengthened our faith and gave us deep courage.

One morning, as I was putting together a list of people I wanted to invite to pray with us, I remembered Russell had an old friend, Wendell Burton, who worked in Joel Osteen's church in Houston. I contacted Wendell to ask him to please pray for Russell, and to say how much Dodie's book had inspired us on our own journey.

Not only did he agree to be part of our prayer network, Wendell told Dodie about us! (Today she is in her 80s, and is in charge of the healing ministry at Lakewood Church.)

The very next day, we received an email from Dodie saying: "Be healed in Jesus' name!" It brought such joy and strength to our hearts.

> In one of Charles Schulz's beloved "Peanuts" cartoons,
> Lucy demands that Linus change TV channels,
> then threatens him with her fist if he doesn't.
> "What makes you think you can walk right in here and take over?" asks Linus.
> "These five fingers," says Lucy. "Individually they are nothing.
> But when I curl them together like this into a single unit,
> they form a weapon that is terrible to behold."
> "What channel do you want?" asks Linus. Then, turning away,
> he looks at his fingers and says:
> "Why can't you guys get organized like that?"

CHAPTER 20
THE NUTRITION STRATEGY

**And ye shall serve the LORD your God, and His blessing will be
on your food and water. I will take sickness away from among you.
— Exodus 23:25-26**

In addition to prayer, nutrition became another key strategy we used to help us defeat the cancer. As we look back, we marvel again at the wisdom of our friends and at God's perfect timing.

In June, after the tumor was discovered, our friend Janet told us of a nutritional approach that had been helping her of debilitating chronic conditions that had afflicted her for more than 20 years. Janet had discovered a nutritional consultant and author named Doug Kaufman.

As she read Doug's book, *The Fungus Link*,[3] and began following his regimen, we witnessed how her energy, mood, weight, pain levels, and resistance to certain food allergies all improved.

The Link Between Fungus and Cancer

Kaufman suggests there are strong links between the presence of fungus in our bodies and many debilitating diseases, including cancer.

Kaufman's website (see the List of Resources at the end), features testimonials of many users of his Phase One Diet being healed of chronic diseases. Between those stories and Janet's transformation, we got very interested and began devouring his materials.

---

3   Kaufman, D. A. (2005). *The Fungus Link, An Introduction to Fungal Disease Including the Initial Phase One Diet*. Rockwall: Mediatrition.

As we delved in, the Kaufman approach made a lot of sense. Although we were already nutrition-conscious and led healthy lifestyles, we began eliminating certain foods completely from our lives, and focused on healthier alternatives.

It felt very empowering to be taking tangible steps in the physical realm, actively combating the cancer instead of just waiting to receive medical treatments. We were also excited that this regimen would help boost Russell's immune system at a time when he was under enormous stress.

To support Russ, I chose to also follow the Kaufman diet. It not only made our meal preparations easier, but offered me many health benefits as well. We were to stick faithfully to the Phase One Diet for the next year, and many of its principles have since become a way of life for us.

Dietary Changes

The following summary of this comprehensive approach is too brief to be prescriptive, but some of the big changes included:

- Eating only organic foods;
- Eliminating sugar completely, as well as honey, agave, maple syrup, molasses, etc. (Cancer feeds on sugar);
- Avoiding popular grains like wheat, corn and white rice that can be full of cancer-causing fungal poisons called mycotoxins (because of the way they are stored);
- Eliminating fruits high in fructose;
- Eating approximately 80 percent vegetables, as well as approved fruits carbs and grains, and 20 percent protein.
- Juicing and drinking delicious combinations of fresh vegetables (especially dark green leafy ones) and select fruits daily;
- Increasing our intake of nuts and seeds, such as almonds, walnuts, cashews, as well as hemp, chia and sunflower seeds.
- Eliminating coffee, tea, and dairy products.

(For a complete list of recommended vegetables, animal protein and other edibles, please consult Kaufman's writings on the Phase One Diet.)

Visible Improvements

Within a few weeks, we both began to feel stronger and have better digestion. Russell's complexion turned from a grayish-white to a healthy pink. He also experienced two other visible improvements:

1. A stubborn black fungus that had lived for *years* under one of Russ's toenails began to grow out, and eventually disappeared.
2. Long-consistent aches in Russell's feet subsided noticeably.

We couldn't help but hope that, if his exterior was showing such tangible progress, there might be wonderful healing also happening on the inside. We dared not get too optimistic, but we certainly felt encouraged, and physically quite energized.

Additional Resources

Our research also included several other books and documentaries (see List of Resources). Two documentaries, "Food Inc." and "Forks Over Knives" in particular, also contain a wealth of wisdom.

On a personal note, I weaned myself off a sugar addiction that would have probably caused me problems down the road. I also enjoyed the added benefit of dropping about 10 pounds.

Exercise and Environment

Exercise continued to play a big part in our lives, to help us manage stress, stay strong, and feel vital. To keep a positive home environment and hopeful state of mind, we also listened to worship music or uplifting sermons during our workouts.

While our days were extremely focused and disciplined, we also pursued our normal activities. Nobody except those we told would have ever known we were in a fight for Russell's life.

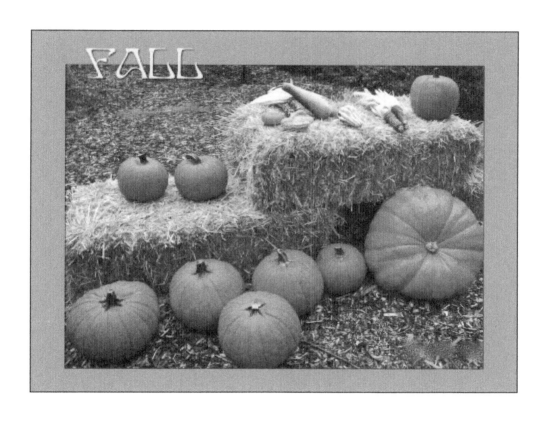

CHAPTER 21

Mixed News

So do not fear , for I am with you; do not be dismayed,
for I am your God; I will strengthen you and help you;
I will uphold you with my righteous right hand.
— Isaiah 41:10

Summer came and went. It had been filled with prayer marathons, nutritional disciplines, spiritual counseling, and our own personal devotions. Finally, our appointment in September arrived.

Russ and I checked into USC's Keck Medical Center at 7:30 a.m. His procedure, with a full anesthetic, was scheduled for 11 a.m. As I sat by his bedside, the hours ticked by. We talked, prayed, read, and dreamed about the future. We were full of faith. "It will all be over soon," we told each other.

Around 1 p.m., the nurse informed us our specialist was running late, due to unexpected complications with another surgery. Russell was quite tired, so I left him to nap and met up with our friends Carmen and Craig.

Once again, they'd come to support Russ and me; they were in the busy waiting area. It was filled with families, TV monitors airing talk shows, and coffee tables messy with magazines.

Carmen and Craig were great company, but I felt tense; I let them do most of the talking while I prayed quietly in my spirit.

The Moment Arrives

Finally, around 5:30 p.m., Russell's surgeon stepped into the waiting room looking for me. By now, I'd been waiting seven hours, though, truthfully, we'd been waiting all summer.

Wearing his blue scrubs and American flag bandana, our Norris urologist announced with a smile: "He's completely healed."

My heart *exploded!* We'd been praying for three months to hear those exact same words!

Thrilled as I was, I had to quickly pull back my emotions. Something told me he was not referring to the cancer, but rather that Russell had recovered well from his bruising tumor surgery in June.

I was right.

"It all looks good," the doctor said, referring to the tissue samples he had just taken. "He's healed well, but we really won't know until we get the biopsy results." Then, turning away, he said: "Call me in a week."

And that was it. After three months of waiting and battle, just one minute of conversation.

I felt relief and fear... hope and uncertainty... joy and frustration. Russell's bladder had recovered well from his first surgery, but the real story lay in what was happening in the tissues.

So, more waiting ahead... no resting at base camp... the climb was not over. The week crept by.

CHAPTER 22
THE CALL

The LORD is close to the brokenhearted, and
saves those who are crushed in spirit.
— Psalm 34:18

The afternoon we were supposed to phone the doctor, Russell was tied up at work. So I made the call alone.

"Two out of four biopsies tested positive for cancer," he reported.

I fell back in my chair, just reeling.

"One is near where the tumor had been, and the other is on the right side of the bladder."

I sat frozen.

"The malignancy is on the surface, but this cancer is wanting to get out," he continued. "We recommend six weeks of localized BCG vaccines as treatment, and then we have to do more biopsies."

Hardly able to talk, I mumbled a few questions about logistics and hung up. Staggering under the weight of this crushing reality, I cried out to God for wisdom and strength.

How was I going to tell Russell? Exactly how *much* should I tell him? Would he buckle under the news? Would

> I will instruct you and teach you
> in the way you should go;
> I will counsel you and watch over you.
> -Psalm 32:8

he feel God had let him down? Had our prayer sessions and nutrition regimens been futile?

I rehearsed my speech for hours, and asked God to please prepare the way.

Breaking the News

When Russell got home, we sat down. I broke the news as gently as I could. He listened bravely and then the hard reality hit. We both sat in silence.

After some time, Russell looked at me.

"The cancer is on the surface," he said. "We can now finally begin the BCG treatments. I'm already healing internally—my toe fungus is gone. We're going to beat this!"

Oh, the relief! A huge weight lifted off me! I thanked the Lord over and over for Russell's response.

I told him we would shoulder the burden together. We would keep the faith that this was just another milestone on the road to victory. Hand in hand we would take the next step forward, and the next, and the next, trusting that God was going before us and preparing the way.

We agreed that we were already halfway up the mountain. There was no turning back now.

CHAPTER 23

A FRESH WIND

Hope is the thing with feathers that perches in the soul,
and sings the tune without words, and never stops at all.
— Emily Dickinson

It was late September when the treatments began. Early every Friday, Russell drove to USC Norris for a vaccine of BCG. Each session lasted about 15 minutes.

While he was undergoing treatment, I hosted a prayer-conference call with five or six friends. They prayed with me for God to anoint the BCG and make it exceedingly effective for Russell's healing. I believe these prayers were mighty on his behalf.

The BCG Approach

In some countries, BCG is used as a vaccine to provide protection against tuberculosis. But in the U.S., it's also used to treat early-stage bladder cancer and prevent recurrences.

The BCG fluid is administered to the bladder via a catheter inserted into the urethra. The procedure is apparently a bit painful as the BCG moves through the prostate.

Thankfully the process takes only a few minutes. The patient must then hold the liquid for two hours before releasing it through the urine.

The bladder recognizes the BCG as a foreign substance, and reacts by becoming inflamed. The inflammation, in turn, stimulates the bladder's own immune response. And thus the bladder "fights back" to destroy foreign and toxic elements—in this case, the cancer cells.

Opinions vary as to the success rates of this BCG therapy. Some suggest it offers a 50- to 60-percent chance of beating cancer. So our surgeon's prognosis to me in June—where he gave the BCG approach only a 25- to 30-percent chance of success—was deeply discouraging. But perhaps his prognosis was because of the toughness of the type of cancer with which we were dealing.

These uncertain odds are what kept me researching other options that might complement the BCG therapy, and thus increasing Russell's chances of healing.

On the bright side, at least we weren't going to be subjected to conventional chemotherapy, which is so destructive to *both* good *and* bad cells, as well as having other debilitating side effects.

The Always-Wonderful Blessing of Friends

As I continued sleuthing in search of other complementary approaches to healing, God used our Christian friends to help direct our next steps.

I had confided my pain and anguish to an old friend who lived in Cambridge, Massachusetts. I'd had the privilege of leading her to the Lord, and we spoke almost weekly by phone.

One day, she saw a television spot—in *Massachusetts!*—about a Christian medical facility in Orange County—*California!*—that specialized in alternative therapies for treating cancer. We both found this dislocated commercial so unusual, it caught our attention: *Could God be in this?*

> I do not wish to treat friendships daintily, but with the roughest courage. When they are real, they are not glass threads or frost-work, but the solidest thing in the world.
> — Ralph Waldo Emerson

I researched the Cancer Center for Hope online, and became captivated by its team and approach. Their success stories—with all types of cancers using nontoxic, pain-free treatments—were especially impressive.

Their website (see List of Resources) also openly acknowledged the work of the Holy Spirit in the healing process! To me, that was quite irresistible.

Several lengthy phone conversations followed, along with exchanges of Russell's CT scans and medical reports. Finally, the Cancer Center team expressed confidence in being able to make a positive contribution to Russell's healing.

I excitedly scheduled an appointment to meet with them. Though more than an hour away from us by car on congested freeways, at least their Irvine branch was in Southern California. God's remarkable provision, once again.

CHAPTER 24
SHARING THE SECRET

If you live to be a hundred, I want to live to be

a hundred minus one day, so I never have to live without you.

— A.A. Milne, in *Winnie the Pooh*

Now that this other promising option had surfaced, I felt the Holy Spirit nudge me: It was time to tell Russell that our USC Norris surgeon gave the BCG only a 25- to 30-percent chance of success.

Russell was absolutely devastated by the news.

"You were right not to tell me back in June," he said. "I would have caved. I can't believe you have carried this burden all these months."

"I did tell Carol, [my sister] and my women's prayer group," I confided. "That's also why I wanted those private sessions with Murray... and you know I met with Pastor Jeff and Patsy. They've all been praying for you—and God has strengthened me."

"Still," Russell said. "Wow."

I told him: "The doctors don't have that last word, darlin'. God does."

"And I know God is going to heal me," he said full of defiant faith.

"I do too!" I exclaimed. "And these treatments might be part of His strategy."

"I believe they are," he said. "And so are the prayers and the diet."

"I completely agree," I told him. "But for the treatments to be successful, you now do need to be aware of the stakes, so you can fully participate."

"With my schedule, how am I going to fit in driving to Orange County and back for treatments?" he said anxiously.

"What if *I* do the driving?" I proposed. "That way you can nap and keep your strength up."

"Man," he said. "It's going to be intense."

"But worth it," I assured him—and needing desperately to believe it myself.

CHAPTER 25
REVIVAL OF THE HEART

I will say of the LORD, He is my fortress and my refuge,

my God in Whom I trust.

— Psalm 91:2

The next morning, when Russell awoke, a dark despair had gripped his heart. I understood the reaction. Up until now he'd been so incredibly brave, so full of faith, so fully committed to every healing approach.

I also knew only too well the crushing weight of those gruesome statistics. When I first heard them, they had brought me to my knees.

I gave Russell some space to process.

In my mind we had reason to hope. The bladder had not developed any other tumors over the summer, and while the cancer was still there and more prevalent than we'd expected, it was on the muscle's surface and in the early stages—as far as we could tell.

I fought to stay positive for both of us, knowing God was fully aware of these developments. Russell's shock and dismay were to be expected. But *now* we had medical treatments and therapies that would help us in the fight—and the Lord's promises to us were still true, whether Russell could believe them this day or not.

We *would* get through this.

Finding Strength in the Lord

Russell sat at the Lord's feet that day, letting the Scriptures wash over him —one hour, two hours, three...

We talked. We reasoned. We prayed.

He found comfort, strength and courage in God's Word. Over and over, I read from key Psalms and other Scriptures that held some of God's greatest promises.

"This is what's true," I reminded us. "God will not fail us."

Gradually, as the Holy Spirit worked on his heart, Russell began to revive. By the end of the day, he had regained his strength and was ready to resume the fight. Once again, he trusted God for his complete healing.

He was back!

CHAPTER 26

An Oasis of Hope

Everything that is done in the world is done by hope.
— Martin Luther

Unlike the hustle and bustle of a hospital, the Cancer Center for Hope (formerly called Oasis of Hope USA), the alternative treatment facility in Irvine, was quite peaceful. Worship music wafted softly overhead as we walked in. Images of serene gardens and Mediterranean seaside villas decorated the beige walls.

Past the entryway, a spacious main room was filled with half-a-dozen large, brown, upholstered armchairs arranged in a semicircle, and facing a giant television. Filling its screen were aerial sweeps of beautiful mountains, waterfalls and wildlife, together with inspirational Scripture verses. More special armchairs were lined up on a side wall.

It was 8 a.m. when we arrived. By midmorning, the big room would be full of seated patients getting their various treatments.

An Alternative Universe

We were greeted by friendly staff, who led us on a tour of many rooms—all fitted with state-of-the-art equipment, each one specially designed for various kinds of alternative therapies.

It was hard not to be amazed by these remarkable machines that offered nontoxic, pain-free treatments, designed to meet the individual healing needs of each patient.

All the approaches were new to us. They included Hyperbaric Oxygen Therapy, Vitamin-C Therapy, Class-IV Laser Therapy, and Pulsed Electromagnetic Field Therapy (details ahead), as well as several others.

In addition to these integrated therapies, the center also offered spiritual counseling and nutrition programs.

The facility was started by Dr. Francisco Contreras, a cancer pioneer internationally recognized for combining conventional and alternative cancer therapies with emotional and spiritual counseling. We learned the Center was also one of the world's leading research institutions in the treatment of cancer. Dr. Contreras also runs an international hospital in Tijuana, Mexico, where he treats patients from more than 60 countries with state-of-the-art integrative therapies.

Our Customized Treatment

After the tour, we met with one of the doctors for a lengthy consultation. He did a careful review of Russell's records, and as we spoke at length, this doctor proved quite knowledgeable in the world of alternative therapies.

At the end, he expressed optimism that several of their treatments could help increase Russ's chances of beating this cancer. The Center had a strong track record of success stories, so we could not help but feel encouraged! We had come in search of enhanced options, and were finding precisely that.

Personalized Mix of Treatments

A short time later, the doctor gave us a customized menu of recommended treatments. The list was very robust, and took us aback.

> Commit to the Lord whatever you do, and your plans will succeed.
> — Proverbs 16:3

We carefully studied the benefits of each approach, and ultimately settled on four out of ten integrated therapies that we felt would likely yield the best results—and that we could afford.

Budgets were a very real consideration, because our health insurance would not cover this kind of treatment.

It is a sad fact of our times that healthcare has become such a huge, complicated business one has to be very shrewd, cautious and wise in pursuit of the best medical solutions.

All Systems Go

Prior to committing, we checked with USC Norris to ensure that these alternative treatments would not conflict with our BCG therapy. Thankfully, they gave us the green light. Feeling reassured, we committed to the alternative treatments with the Cancer Center.

For the next two months, our schedules became very intense. Every Tuesday and Thursday we would drive from Los Angeles to Irvine—42.5 miles each way—for four hours of alternative treatments. And on Friday mornings Russ would head to USC Norris for the BCG treatments.

It's a testament to God's grace and sustaining power that Russell was able to keep working during this entire time, never missing a beat although, obviously, the hectic schedule was tiring.

In God's divine providence, I was still in transition between jobs. This allowed me to be at Russ's side every step of the way, helping meet his needs and lighten the load.

It was obvious to me that God had orchestrated the break for such a time as this. I was also certain that when it was all over, He would open the next professional door for me, which is exactly what happened.

> **With my last breath I'll exhale my love for you.**
> **I hope it's a cold day, so you can see what you meant to me.**
> **— Jarod Kintz**

CHAPTER 27

ALTERNATIVE THERAPIES

Anyone who has faith in me will do what I have been doing.

He will do even greater things than these, because

I am going to the Father.

— Jesus, in John 14:12

The following is an overview of the alternative therapies we received at The Cancer Center.

Hyperbaric Oxygen Therapy (HBOT)

Cancer likes certain kinds of environments in which to grow. A low-oxygen environment is one of cancer's favorites. Conversely, it's believed that an oxygen-rich environment may prove hostile to malignancies.

HBOT is a medical procedure wherein patients breathe 100-percent-pure oxygen while resting inside pressurized chambers. This process increases the amount of oxygen carried in the blood, and stimulates the release of substances that promote healing.[4]

Scuba divers have used this method for decompression since the 1930s, when the military developed it for deep-sea diving and aeronautic purposes. Today, HBOT is also being used to treat up to a dozen other conditions, including autism, wounds associated with radiation exposure, and cerebrovascular diseases.

---

4   Oasis of Hope. *Hyperbaric Oxygen Treatment.* (n.d.) Retreived September 26, 2012 from <u>www. oasisofhopeusa.com</u>.

It should be noted, however, that conclusive evidence as to its effectiveness is still pending.[5]

HBOT chambers come in various styles. Russell's looked like a long hollow capsule. The inside contained a narrow mattress, and a window along the length of the side. Once Russell lay comfortably inside, the technicians slowly pressurized the chamber and pumped in the oxygen.

During these 90-minute sessions, Russ was able to sleep, listen to music, watch a video, or pray. Most of the sessions, he'd just nap and feel great afterwards!

Vitamin C Therapy

Doctors have been studying the cancer-killing effects of high doses of vitamin C since the 1970s, beginning with Nobel-Prize-winning scientist Linus Pauling.

Since then, the National Institutes of Health, the National Cancer Institute, and the Food and Drug Administration—in addition to numerous published case reports from other medical facilities[6]—have confirmed that repeated high doses of intravenous vitamin C can cause tumors to regress.

Further, the Center contends that when the intravenous vitamin C is combined with oxygen, the oxygen converts to hydrogen peroxide, sending an even deadlier blow into malignant areas, while leaving normal cells unharmed. This is unheard of with the conventional treatments, such as chemotherapy, that simultaneously target *both* cancerous *and* healthy cells.[7]

After each HBOT treatment, Russ would sit comfortably in an upholstered chair while two full bags of vitamin C were administered intravenously. He experienced no discomfort, and was able to read or catch up on work during these times.

---

5   Mayo Clinic. *Hyperbaric Oxygen Therapy.* Retrieved September 26, 2012 from www.mayoclinic.com/health/hyperbaric-oxygen-therapy/my00829.

6   Oasis of Hope. *Vitamin C* video retrieved September 26, 2012 from www.oasisofhope.com/vitamin-c.php.

7   Oasis of Hope. *Vitamin C* video retrieved September 26, 2012 from www.oasisofhope.com/vitamin-c.php.

Class-IV Laser Therapy

The Center uses Class IV Laser therapy in conjunction with Vitamin C therapy and HBOT. Laser therapy is FDA approved.

The laser's infrared light (measured in watts) is delivered via a hand held "flashlight" device that is gently rubbed over the surface of the malignant area(s). The laser light penetrates deeply into the damaged and poorly oxygenated tissue. This causes the blood and lymphatic vessels to dilate making the target area hyper-receptive to the vitamin C and oxygen therapy being delivered via the blood supply.[8]

While vitamin C and oxygen help strengthen the patient's immune system, the combination is toxic to cancer and helps hinder its growth.[9]

Laser therapy also increases circulation of the lymph system, which aids in the elimination of toxins. This cleansing is a critically important aspect of the healing process.[10]

In Russell's case, the tumor surgery had left swelling and trauma in his bladder tissue. During his weekly treatments, the hand held laser device was gently swiped over his bladder area for fifteen minutes per session. He found it soothing and painless.

Pulsed Electromagnetic Field Therapy (PEMF)

Pulsed Electromagnetic Field Therapy (PEMF) therapy was approved by the FDA in 1982 as an aid in the healing of bone fractures.[11] It also has been used in Europe for more than 30 years to help heal soft-tissue wounds, alleviate pain and increase range of motion.[12]

---

8   Oasis of Hope. *Class-IV Laser Therapy* retrieved September 27, 2012 from www.oasisofhopeusa.com.

9   Oasis of Hope. *Class-IV Laser Therapy* retrieved September 27, 2012 from www.oasisofhopeusa.com.

10   Oasis of Hope. *Class-IV Laser Therapy* retrieved September 27, 2012 from www.oasisofhopeusa.com.

11   PEMF.US. *Peer Reviewed Scientific Studies on the Effects of Magnetics on Physical Ailments.* Retrieved September 29, 2012 from www.pemf.us/study.html.

12   PEMF.US. *Peer Reviewed Scientific Studies on the Effects of Magnetics on Physical Ailments.* Retrieved September 29, 2012 from www.pemf.us/study.html.

This reparative treatment converts a magnetic field into a series of tiny electrical pulses that are applied to the injured tissue.

Studies show that healthy tissue has an electric potential of approximately 110mV (millivolts), whereas tumorous tissue has a much-lower electric potential (approximately 25mV)[13]

The Center also uses PEMF therapy to battle cancer in conjunction with Vitamin C therapy and/or HBOT treatments. It is believed that application of the PEMF electrical pulses to the malignant areas interrupts (or scrambles) the normal electrical communication between cancer cells, thus inhibiting tumor growth. It also provides cells with an energy boost that helps restore them to health and aid in eliminating toxins.[14]

Quadruple Punch

Russell had weekly, 6-minute PEMF treatments after the HBOT, Vitamin-C and Class-IV K Laser therapies. Administration of these four treatments took about four hours each visit. Thankfully, Russell's only side effect was a little fatigue. But this was more from having to squeeze the visits into a hectic work schedule, rather than from the therapies themselves.

If anything, Russ's treatments at the Center were fortifying and boosted his immune system.

His complementary treatments of BCG (Bacillus Calmette-Guerin) at USC Norris were also about 15 minutes each. Though BCG does have *potential* side effects such as flu-like symptoms and fever, Russell experienced none of these.[15]

As a result, he kept up his normal schedule and life throughout this entire season of therapies—a miracle and blessing beyond words.

---

13   Oasis of Hope. *Class-IV Laser Therapy* retrieved September 28, 2012 from www.oasisofhopeusa.com.

14   Oasis of Hope. *Class-IV Laser Therapy* retrieved September 28, 2012 from www.oasisofhopeusa.com.

15   American Cancer Society. *Intravesical Therapy for Bladder Cancer* retrieved July 9, 2012 from www. cancer.org/cancer/bladdercancer/detailedguide/bladder-cancer-treating-intravesical-therapy.

(PLEASE NOTE: We carefully and prayerfully chose our combination of treatments to assist with Russell's particular cancer. We do not suggest or imply that this exact combination of therapies is a healing formula for someone else's condition. Cancer treatment should be tailored to every person's individual needs.)

I will strengthen you and help you;
I will uphold you with my righteous right hand.
— Isaiah 41:10

CHAPTER 28
A MUCH-NEEDED BREAK

Consider it all joy, my brothers, when you face various trials,
for you know the testing of your faith produces perseverance.
— James 1:3

I t was mid-October when we finally finished our six weeks of BCG and alternative therapies.

Now, for the treatments to run their course, we had to wait six more weeks before Russ could submit to a second biopsy on December 21 with another full anesthetic.

However, because of the holidays, we would not get the results before Christmas. We would have to wait until January to learn of any progress.

Waiting is a hard lesson—and it never became easy. But, as we had done so many times throughout this trial, we turned to the Scriptures for strength.

> **But those who hope in the LORD will renew their strength.**
> **They will soar on wings like eagles;**
> **they will run and not grow weary,**
> **they will walk and not be faint.**
> **— Isaiah 40:31**

So many biblical leaders went through their seasons of testing—and indescribably worse than ours:

David battled Saul for years, until his rightful time to assume the throne; Jacob waited 14 years instead of seven for Rachel to become his bride; Hannah suffered decades of humiliation and loneliness before the birth of Samuel; Abraham and

Sarah waited 25 years for the fulfillment of Isaac, the son of promise... and these are just a few!

Though our trials could not compare to these heroes of the faith, it was nevertheless our personal time of testing; we found ourselves *quite* emotionally exhausted.

Russell's birthday was coming up. So we decided to take a much-needed break and rest for a few days.

A travel-agent friend had told me about a sleepy-but-artsy community in Jalisco, Mexico, on the shores of a big lake. We both agreed it sounded perfect.

Once again, we had no idea what lay ahead.

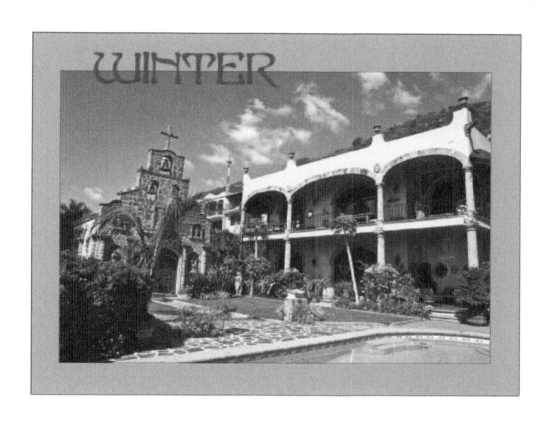

CHAPTER 29

A Surreal Vacation

Un país donde el surrealismo es vida
y la muerte es una santa hecha de metal y resina.
A country where surrealism is life
and death is a saint made of metal and resin.
— Jose Gil Olmos

I had made our reservations before we found out about the murders.

Our destination was Ajijic, Mexico, a small lakeside resort noted for its warm weather, cobblestone streets, art scene, and restaurants. While scanning the local online news for fun things to do, I learned that only six months earlier, rival drug gangs had massacred 18 young locals and strewn their dismembered remains along the town's hills and roads.

The quiet town of 15,000, normally sheltered from drug violence, was terrorized for weeks. Eventually things settled down; however, there was a new awareness that their old way of life had suffered an irretrievable blow.

As Russ and I grappled with whether to scrap the entire trip, we learned the violence had erupted over transport routes primarily among the drug gangs themselves. Further research also reassured us that hundreds of retired Americans lived in Ajijic. So, desperately needing a break, we decided to go.

Unique

Mexico has always been a country of dramatic contrasts and contradictions. On our taxi ride from the Guadalajara airport to our bed and breakfast in Ajijic, we passed clusters of shantytowns coexisting near luxury homes and modern malls. These two realities are a common sight and part of the country's socioeco-nomic tapestry.

Spectacular properties in Mexico often hide behind high walls. This proved true for us. As we stepped out of our cab onto the narrow cobblestone street and through the gates of our bed and breakfast, we stepped into an absolute paradise!

Lush terraced gardens, winding paths hugged by plants flowering in purple and pink, gurgling fountains, stone sculptures, walls painted in burgundy and gold—all enveloped our senses with a sensuous embrace.

Our B&B was actually a European-style villa of breathtaking beauty.

Its name was Villa del Angel, and from its cushion-filled patios we could admire its sculptured landscape, turquoise pool, gray stone chapel, and the most spectacular hillside view of Lake Chapala (Mexico's largest freshwater lake, 50 miles long and 15 miles across).

Our suite was the highest room on the property. We climbed a winding brick staircase flanked by ironwork frothing with crimson bougainvillea. Our room was an apartment-sized suite with a fireplace, beamed ceilings, sitting area, and a balcony boasting a panoramic view of both the town and the lake. We were in heaven!

A Hint of Mystery

"You can stay in any of the other rooms if you prefer," the owner told us. "You're the only guests."

"Why are we the only guests?" I asked. "It's gorgeous here!"

"Oh," she answered nonchalantly, "people are still scared."

As we would soon find out, that was only *part* of the story.

That evening, we enjoyed a scrumptious dinner of tamarind chicken at one of the town's 20 restaurants. Having been warned not to walk the streets at night, we had a taxi drop us at the villa's back entrance, so the cabbie didn't have to drive up the killer cobblestoned hill to the front gate.

Unfortunately, by now it was dark. Though we fumbled for several minutes, our keys wouldn't open the lock. Suddenly, before we could even protest, our driver scrambled up and over the gate and opened it from the other side. Then, leaping back in his cab, he quickly drove away, leaving us with our jaws open.

"Ah, Mexico," I smiled, stunned but grateful.

An Unexpected Twist

We entered in and began the slow climb up the villa's lower garden. It was dark and we were unfamiliar with this part of the property. We looked for recognizable landmarks as we progressed. Strangely, none were to be found. In fact, this property didn't look like the villa at all.

The truth suddenly hit us: *We were on the wrong property!*

"Great! Breaking and entering—on our vacation!" I exclaimed.

Scrambling like two teenagers to escape before the owners, dogs, house guards, police—or all four—discovered us, we soon found ourselves exactly where we shouldn't have been in Mexico: Stranded alone at night in a dark back alley.

Welcome to Ajijic!

Though I'd spent many happy years growing up in Mexico, times had changed. I no longer felt as safe, especially in a town I did not know.

Fortunately my Spanish was still good, so we walked up the road and I asked a young couple necking in a doorway if they knew where our street was. The young man pointed, but it led to a dead end.

"Ah, Mexico," I commented again. Ruefully, this time.

We walked back in the opposite direction till we reached a wider road with streetlights. Not having anticipated this evening's on-foot excursion, with every step I now felt my high-heeled ankle boots slipping and sliding over the rugged cobblestones.

We finally found a small shop still open. The young girl inside sat on a plastic chair under a naked light bulb, flanked by shelves filled with boxed candy, detergent, and soft drinks.

I asked politely if she'd call us a taxi to take us back to the villa. She said we were closer than we thought and pointed the way. So (*perhaps* a little prematurely), we decided it would be faster to walk.

The trek involved a steep climb up several long cobblestoned blocks. It was not a great part of town, and as we passed by, several stragglers and street kids stared questioningly at the obviously-out-of-place tourist couple.

Moving briskly, we suddenly encountered a gang of eight young men, in their twenties, lurking on a corner. They all turned to study us.

"Don't make eye contact," I advised Russell.

Suddenly, out of nowhere, a dull yellow 1960s Oldsmobile crept up slowly behind us, then came alongside so the driver could check us out.

"Just keep going," whispered Russell. We ignored the car and kept walking.

The car then swerved in front of us, cutting us off. Our hearts pounding, but refusing to show fear, we kept moving forward, Russell to the left around the car and I to the right.

Next, the killer hill, our final stretch, lay ahead. As we began the climb, our pace considerably slowed. If anyone had wanted to nab us from behind, we were easy pickings at this point.

We prayed for safety every step of the way, just certain we were being watched.

Breathing hard and leg muscles stinging, we finally made it to the top of our hill. Oh, happy sight! There was the villa gate—and the key fit! We'd made it home!

Nocturne Serenade

Within minutes we were curled up in our luxurious bed, dozing off—when suddenly BOOM! Boom! Boom, boom! Boom, boom, boom! Boom, BOOM!

"What is that?!?" I exclaimed, bolting up. "Fireworks?"

"Explosives," groaned Russell, rolling over and pulling a pillow over his head.

Seconds later, a loud brass band began its "bumpa, bumpa, bumpa, bumpa"! Trumpets, drums, cymbals—and an inebriated singer—belted out an off-key *corrido* (country ballad) through distorted speakers.

Given that our villa was atop a hill, the sound traveled into our bedroom like a laser beam. To add to the cacophony, the town's church bells rang like clockwork, every hour on the hour. This delirium went on *all night long.*

It felt like a conspiracy!

In the morning, we uncovered the truth. As it turns out, we had arrived smack in the middle of the pueblo's annual "fiestas" honoring their patron saint. There would be festivities, music, explosives, fireworks, and church bells from sundown to sunup, for 14 days straight!

So the *real* reason the villa had no other guests wasn't just the drug wars, it was the fiestas! Most of the American residents in Ajijic had escaped to Puerto Vallarta till after Christmas.

Thus we had arrived in paradise, but sleep would elude us. It was a "minor detail" the villa owner had neglected to share.

It had all become even more vivid: Mexico wasn't just a land of contrasts—it was just plain surreal.

Blessed by Art

We cut short our Ajijic stay. We took a taxi to Tlaquepaque, a suburb of Guadalajara—Mexico's second-largest city, and famous for its colonial beauty.

Here we stayed at a charming inn called Quinta San Jose, just one block away from the cultural center that overflows with spectacular art: paintings, sculptures, folk art, embroidered linens, and leather goods. The center also boasts a great selection of international restaurants.

Mexico's art is robust, daring, and energizing, and we found our spirits lifted by it. Strolling under the warm sun, we admired the creative blend of Spanish Colonial and modern architecture, and relaxed enough to buy a few beautiful items for our home. Their purchase spurred optimism in our hearts.

Viva México

Sad to say, a good night's sleep eluded us in Tlaquepaque as well. Our lovely suite was right off the swimming pool and hotel guests indulged in Happy Hour with splashing gusto till about 4 a.m.

Yet despite these trials, Mexico's beauty and hospitality did provide a welcome reprieve from our personal stress. We returned to Los Angeles surprisingly refreshed.

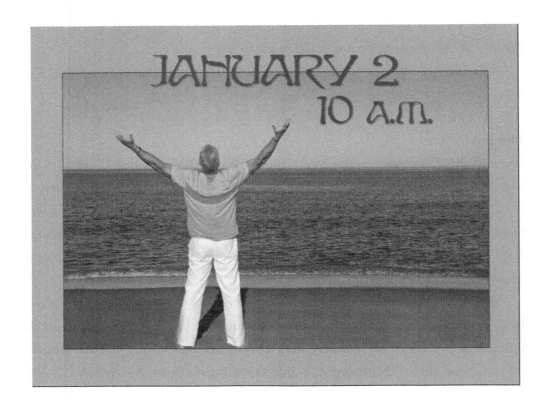

CHAPTER 30
VICTORY AT LAST

**Victory at all costs, victory in spite of all terror,
victory however long and hard the road may be.
— Winston Churchill**

Stepping through the front door of our lovely home, we were greeted by our four cats. They were overjoyed to see us. A short while later, we all curled up in our own comfortable bed and Russ and I got the first good night's sleep in two weeks!

January 2nd arrived soon after. At 10 a.m. we phoned the USC Norris Cancer Center to get the lab results of Russell's biopsy.

We were bracing ourselves for the news. Half of me was hoping for the best, the other half didn't dare hope. The atmosphere was tense. Russell was on one phone receiver. I was on another.

"The tests were negative," said the nurse.

"What do you mean, 'negative'?" asked Russell.

"The tests were all clear," she replied.

"Do you mean 'clear' as in no cancer?" I asked, holding my breath.

"That's right," she said cheerfully. "No cancer. No traces of cancer."

"Praise God!" shouted Russell.

"Yay!" giggled the nurse.

I was speechless, overwhelmed.

Just like that, in the blink of an eye, our trial was suddenly over. There was "no cancer, no traces of cancer." We'd been set free!

We could hardly contain ourselves. We hooped and hollered, hugged and cried. We stared at each other and laughed in disbelief. Our cats thought we had lost our minds.

It had been ten full months, from the first sight of blood in March the previous year to this phone call in January.

> **Surely He will save you from the fowler's snare and from the deadly pestilence. He will cover you with his feathers, and under His wings, you will find shelter.**
> **Psalm 91:3-4**

To be honest, I had mentally prepared to hear that Russ showed some improvement but was not out of the woods yet. The "all clear" seemed too good to be true...but it *was* true!

Except for regular check ups every six months, we'd just be handed a new lease on life. Russell was cancer free! It was all wonderful and joyous...and the moment was charged with emotion.

CHAPTER 31

TO GOD BE THE GLORY

**Praise the LORD, O my soul; all my inmost being, praise His holy name.
Praise the LORD, O my soul, and forget not all His benefits
—Who forgives all your sins and heals all your diseases,
Who redeems your life from the pit and crowns you
with love and compassion,
Who satisfies your desires with good things
so that your youth is renewed like the eagle's.
— Psalm 103:1-5**

Though we could now legitimately say we were healed, healthy and whole, the challenge would be to stay that way. That meant being vigilant and disciplined. So, moving forward, our maintenance regime would consist of a mostly plant-based diet, regular exercise and making consistently healthy lifestyle choices—including scheduling more fun and relaxation!

As we look back, we can honestly say we are grateful for the lessons and everything we learned. We now clearly see how from the very beginning, God was behind the scenes orchestrating events. While the cancer was a shock to us and left us feeling out of control, it was no surprise to God.

We're forever grateful that He allowed us to catch the cancer early. Then, despite our panicked confusion about the maze of options and challenges, He guided us to the best doctors and treatments.

He also arranged a parenthesis in my professional career precisely when Russell needed me. Despite the income adjustment, God also provided the financial resources for medical expenses.

To give us courage, God led us to the most outstanding pastors and counselors. Their special gifting helped heal our brokenness, catapult our faith to new heights, and teach us what it really means to trust Him.

To encourage and comfort us, He also blessed us with an outpouring of love and support from our extraordinary community of family and friends who encouraged our hearts, lifted our burdens, and enveloped us with prayers and affection that gave us strength for the climb.

Lastly, we bow down at the feet of Him who made it all possible. We thank God for His Word, the ultimate source of truth and hope which guided us every day, equipped us for battle, and led us to victory.

We are so deeply, eternally, profoundly grateful...to God be the glory!

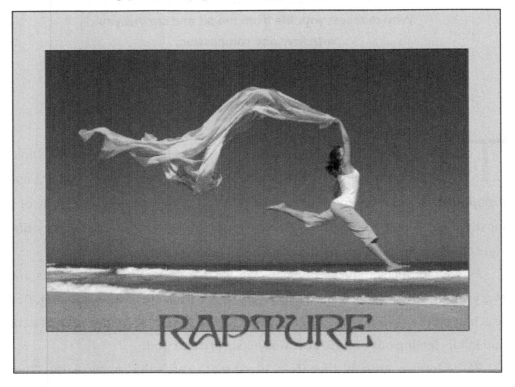

YOU TURNED MY WAILING INTO DANCING.
YOU REMOVED MY SACKCLOTH AND CLOTHED ME WITH JOY.

- PSALM 30:11

(PLEASE NOTE: For those who may be struggling with more advance stages of cancer, the specialists and resources in this book have helped many people make dramatic recoveries. We encourage you to not give up hope and research these options.)

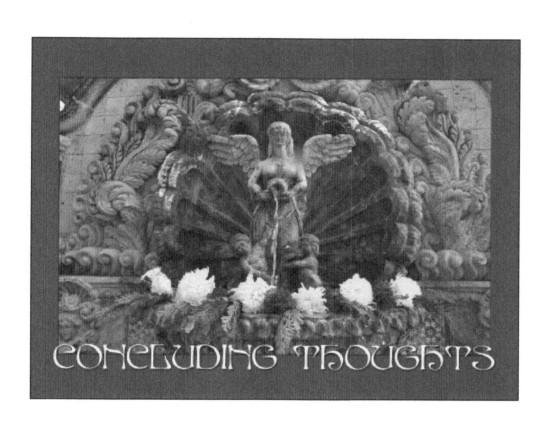

CONCLUDING THOUGHTS

CHAPTER 32
30 Lessons from the Trenches

Praise be to the God and Father of our Lord Jesus Christ,
the Father of all compassion and the God of all comfort,
Who comforts us in all our troubles, so that we can comfort those
in any trouble with the comfort we ourselves have received.
— 2 Corinthians 1:3-4

- God doesn't expect us to be able to see the future. He just asks us to trust Him and to keep moving forward in faith.

- It is not the size of our faith, but the One in Whom we have faith that makes all the difference.

- Faith feeds on the Word of God. Daily time in the Scriptures feeds and equips us with the courage, strength and wisdom needed for the journey.

- Healing journeys are uniquely individual. Find your way *spiritually* through the Scriptures and prayer, *medically* through research and doctors, and *relationally* through your community.

- Ultimately, all healing comes from the Lord—and sometimes He uses doctors and treatments.

- Unforgiveness, fear, sin, etc.—all can be hindrances to healing. Confess, repent and surrender these to God so the Holy Spirit is free to do His work.

- Unless you trust that you're in the best hands, always get a second, third or even fourth medical opinion! Nobody cares about your health or the health of your loved one as much as you. Be prepared to be your own health advocate.

- There are no stupid questions when lives are at stake. Study, research, consult, ask questions, and do not settle until you feel you know what you need to know.

- As a general practicioner once said, "Surgeons like to cut." Before you agree to surgery, be absolutely sure it's the best and *only* way. If there are other alternatives, give them a chance!

- The human body wants to get well and will cooperate with healing measures, so commit to good nutrition and exercise regimens that boost your immune system. Eliminate toxins, and begin building healthy habits for the long term.

- Even when the way is not clear, God is always working behind the scenes working all things out for your good. "Lean not on your own understanding, but in all your ways acknowledge Him, and He will make your paths straight." (Proverbs 3:5).

- Think of ongoing prayer as *spiritual therapy*. Keep a journal of God's promises to you in your situation. Memorize as many of these as possible, then pray them back to God daily.

- As you experience answers these prayers (large and small) write them down. They will encourage your heart and root themselves deeper as you move on through different phases.

- When starting a prayer chain and organizing opportunities for group sessions, be sure and articulate what you believe God is doing in your situation and what your personal goals are so everyone clearly understands and can pray in agreement. Most people sincerely want to help but aren't sure how to pray in really tough circumstances. Focused prayers are very powerful and effective.

- Repeatedly let your prayer partners know how much you appreciate their intercession on your behalf. Real prayer is hard work! Also be sure to keep everyone regularly updated as things evolve.

- It's also important to keep these prayer warriors motivated, so share with them whenever you see answered prayer. Your victory is their victory, too! Good news strengthens everyone's faith and brings glory to God.

- Don't be discouraged or surprised if some people fall away when the battle is longer and harder than they expected. Most people underestimate the fervency and frequency of prayer that are needed to facilitate a break-through in a really tough situation. But *you* must never give up!

- Fasting is a critical component to breakthrough prayer. Ask the Lord to direct what kind and what length of fast He might require of you in your situation. (There is much information out there on different types of fasts.)

- If God wakes you up at odd hours of the night to pray, or similarly burdens you during the day, be quick to respond. It means He has an important insight, instruction or encouragement to equip you, to strengthen you, or to call you to intercede and help win a battle. And, yes, this can mean that sometimes you might be inconvenienced and lose a little sleep!

- In times of trouble, praise and worship are mighty weapons to drive back and defeat the enemies of our soul. Read about Jehoshaphat in 2 Chronicles 20:21, or this passage in 2 Corinthians 10:4: "The weapons we fight with are not the weapons of this world; on the contrary, they have the divine power to demolish strongholds."

- When our hearts are weighed down with anguish, our spirits can still choose to focus on God. In this way, we can rise like an eagle above the pain, know the "peace that surpasses understanding" (Philippians 4:7) and experience how "the joy of the Lord is our strength" (Psalm 28:7).

- You cannot win today's battle with yesterday's strategy. You will need fresh resources for new trials. Ask God for your daily supply. This likely will entail the building of new spiritual muscles, for trials come to "make us mature and complete, lacking nothing" (James 1:4).

- Pray for others. Part of your healing comes from taking your eyes off yourself and lifting up the burdens of others. "He who refreshes others will himself be refreshed" (Proverbs 11:25).

- Stay in community; *never* go it alone. Wisdom and protection come from a multitude of counselors and their support during tough times (Proverbs 24:6).

- Surround yourself with people who have faith in your healing. Avoid those who doubt, mock or dismiss that you can be completely healed.

- Our bladder-cancer-healing journey was not just about us. God blessed us so we could bless others (Genesis 12:3).
- Whatever *you* learn in your journey, share it. Somebody, somewhere needs what you have.
- If you are now cancer-free, God has saved you for a higher purpose. Embrace that fully and step out in faith and in His strength.
- If you do not yet know Jesus, ask Him right now to come into your life, to forgive you for trying to live your life on your own, and invite Him to guide your steps from this moment forward. Then, go tell a genuine Christian about what you have done and let them help you get settled in a church that faithfully teaches the Scriptures. Watch your life take off!
- If you found this book helpful, please tell others who may need it. And may God grant you and all those you love the blessing of living life healed, healthy and whole!

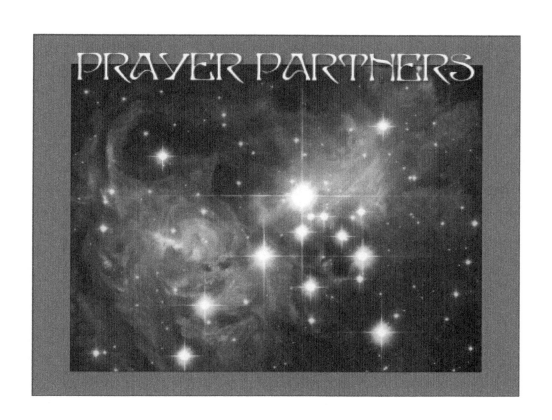

PRAYER PARTNERS

CHAPTER 33

OUR PRAYER PARTNERS SPEAK

Love always protects, always trusts, always hopes, always perseveres.

Love never fails.

— I Corinthians 13:7 & 8

"Watching Russell and Marion go through this was kind of like watching the Olympics. There was that palpable sense that right now everything is on the line. And then the strange feeling of hope mixed with anticipation and anxiety, because you know both of them have spent their lives preparing for this moment.

"It was as if all the quiet times, Bible studies, fellowship, books, and deeds of faith were simply rehearsals for such a time as this. I found myself watching in awe at their humble submission to God as they stepped out of the boat and walked across the water—their faces fixed on God, their hearts set for complete obedience.

"It was truly something to aspire to. It was faith in action."

— Marquis, Pittsburgh, Pennsylvania

"Russell and Marion: Now there's a couple—the perfect match!

"The reaction to his diagnosis was amazing. They went into battle mode with laser focus. When they organized prayer meetings, their house overflowed. Everyone wanted to be there.

"From the beginning I was impressed by the singular belief that Russell would be healed. The faith and love were palpable. People were energized and encouraged by one another, and I was led to fast for Russell. After about six weeks, I woke up one day and believed Russell was healed.

"The thing that touched me most was the deep love these people had for Russell and Marion, and their desire to pray for him. Since his healing, I find myself praying more and with greater conviction. I know others feel the same as they seek out prayer partners, and are emboldened as never before to ask for what previously they would not.

"I believe God used Russell's cancer and healing to demonstrate to those who prayed the powerful results of their united front and His great delight in answering 'yes, yes, yes.'

"Bless you, Russell and Marion; may you enjoy many more years together."
— Janet W., Los Angeles, California

"Not long after renewing my friendship with Russ and getting to know Marion for the first time, his cancer diagnosis arrived. The 'chance' meeting at a restaurant and the subsequent news of his illness soon revealed the fingerprints of a sovereign plan at work.

"Having personally gone through two battles with cancer myself (I am gratefully cancer-free today), I could readily empathize with the daunting struggles Russ and Marion suddenly faced: fear, loss, uncertainty over the best treatments to take, and the challenges to one's faith for God's healing.

"Thankfully, Russ had a tower of faith in Marion, who made it clear from the get-go that there was to be no relenting until the cancer was defeated... and GONE!

"My part became clearer after leading the two of them in a prayer found in a booklet I wrote, titled *More Life! Breaking Free... from the Spirit of Death*. Their reaction was immediate: Fear lifted, hope ensued, and clarity of purposed resumed.

"After sharing that experience with friends, they asked if Embracing Life Ministries (which I direct) might consider doing a *More Life!* seminar for their home group, to get their praying friends on the same page. Of course we agreed. Thus, as this book attests, we all got to play a wonderful part in God's healing of our dear friend and brother. Good news indeed!"

— Jonathan, Pasadena, California

"The courage with which you shared your journey was inspiring. I understand the need for privacy (I've been the sole support for someone journeying with cancer on one occasion), but I have no doubt that if it is possible to open up the journey to family and friends, then the healing can be hastened and the support can be shared... and lessons can be learned.

"The value of the group's love and prayers cannot possibly be underestimated, in my opinion, and you two are proof of this: That a problem shared is no longer a problem, but a journey walked in love."

— Ailsa, Melbourne, Australia

"It was weird how it started—my part of this whole battle for Russell's life, I mean. And it started before anyone—well, anyone except the Lord —even suspected Russell had cancer.

"I was home on a weekend relaxing, sitting in my favorite spot, channel-surfing on the couch with the pillows adjusted just the way I like them for maximum comfort. When all of a sudden, there he was: Doug Kaufman, hosting his show called 'Know the Cause.'

"I was instantly fascinated, and knew this was somebody I needed to listen to. 'The cause' was, according to Kaufman, the dangerous mycotoxins that are produced by various kinds of unfriendly fungi.

"They grow out of control in our bodies because of lots of different problems: our overuse of antibiotics; eating chicken and other meats that are full of antibiotics; wa-a-a-ay too much sugar in our diet (which feeds molds); mold growing unchecked in stored grains; poor diet; and other factors.

"What did Doug say these mycotoxins were the cause of? Everything from athlete's foot to cancer. I didn't have cancer, as far as I knew, but I had had chronic health problems my entire adult life—migraines, chronic digestive problems, chronic fatigue, and others. Doug quoted studies by the most prestigious universities and organizations in the world, and published in the most distinguished journals.

"I started to follow Doug Kaufman's diet guidelines, and pretty soon I began to see results. And as I began to see results and tell about them, Russell and Marion became increasingly interested.

"But they had always eaten what most of us would consider a very healthy diet, and didn't see any great reason to change, although they were happy for me. That is, until they got the report from the doctor: bladder cancer.

"We were all stunned and scared for Russell. But Marion, being who she is, flew into action. She started researching good medical facilities, various approaches available, etc. And she wanted to research diet, too. The problem was, you can find countless gurus on the Internet that support every conceivable diet for cancer. But which one is right? There was no room for error here.

"So I gave her a friendly reminder: What about the Kaufman diet? You've already seen someone getting results from it, and his theories are unquestionably supported by well-documented evidence.

"She enthusiastically embraced it, as did Russell. And as time progressed, and we read and listened more and more, and saw improvements in Russell's body, we became increasingly convinced it was from the Lord. I believe this is one of the means God used to heal Russell.

"The other thing Marion did was to organize prayer groups. Of course, Marion being Marion, and fighting for her husband's life, she did it in a big way.

"Those of us who could be there in person, we went to the Pyles' house for these meetings. Those who couldn't be present but wanted to participate, they were Skyped in on a speaker. Never mind that I couldn't understand a word they said. God could!

"As I review the events of those days, certain images jump out at me: First, approaching those big double doors at the entry to their home. Quite impressive, those doors. I felt I was going to visit a king.

"Then I'd remember I *was* going to visit a King!

"In fact, I was going to visit the King of kings! He would be there and we would petition Him on behalf of one of His beloved subjects. How could He refuse us?

"I remember entering the house and being wrapped in a big bear hug by Russell. If he was afraid, it never showed. He was clearly delighted to see each friend that arrived, and poured out love on us all with his usual abandon. Then, of course, there was Marion, the Lioness, fighting fiercely to save her mate.

"She, too, gave each one a gracious greeting and continued with her preparations, determined to remain focused on the fight, and to encourage the rest of us to join in with all the intensity we could bring to bear. I think the Lord, knowing what Russell was going to face, brought Russell and Marion together as a couple for 'such a time as this.'

"I remember us all sitting in a circle and Marion putting on praise music. I don't remember who the artist was, but as soon as the music started I was overwhelmed with a sense of the Holy Spirit's presence.

"Being touched deeply inside, I began crying. Not wishing to make a scene, I buried my face in my hands and tried to cry silently, so the others' worship would not be disturbed.

"Soon I was doubled over, face in my lap as the music washed over me and the Spirit moved. Other times, people would 'randomly' pray as the Spirit moved them, both in person and on Skype. Then someone would start a worship song and we would all join in. We might stay in our seat, or stand, or go and lay hands on Russell. I guess the only rule was, there weren't any rules.

"Between meetings, Marion would keep us all updated by email. We'd get the ongoing story of challenges and victories, and we'd pray for each new circumstance as it came up. I became convinced that Russell was being healed.

"And over time the good reports began to outnumber the bad reports, and Russell—after a long, hard-fought battle—was pronounced cancer-free. It was a wonderful time of seeing the body of Christ come together to worship and do battle in the Spirit. And by His grace, we were blessed with an amazing victory!"

— Janet C., Los Angeles, California

"I am so grateful to know such wonderful Christians as Russell and Marion. They have been a great support to our ministry in India, and loving friends. When Russell found out he had bladder cancer, they were both working diligently on a fundraiser for India.

"I was very worried about Russell. I felt something serious could be wrong, despite him saying that the doctor said any abnormalities could be from strain to his body from weightlifting. When they found out that it was in fact cancer, immediately the solidarity of their team went into action!

"There are many observations to express, but two that stand out in my mind: first, the prayer meeting that was held. It was so delightful to be a part of it, even though it was only by phone. Second, the fact that despite Russell's being sick, life went on! We stayed at their home twice during this ordeal.

"It was great to be able to engage with people going through so much, and to feel that we are going through it with them. I learned so much about good health, through and through! Thank you, Russell and Marion; and thank You, God, for allowing Russell to stay with us here on earth for many years to come!"

— Amy, Pacifica, California

"It was quite a shock to hear our good friend Russell was stricken with cancer. I think our initial reaction was one of fear and sadness. But the news did something else also: it kicked our faith into overdrive, and got us thinking about Russell instead of ourselves. God began to reveal Himself to us, and others, in new and exciting ways. Yes, it started a rollercoaster of highs and lows, but God was along for the ride.

"How do we describe the journey? It begins with the initial outpouring of prayer and support that is full of hope, emotion and anticipation of instant healing. This is followed by feelings of helpless disappointment when instant healing doesn't come.

"Seeds of doubt begin to fill our minds. Perhaps we didn't pray enough or we didn't pray the right way. Maybe there is some reason for this? Maybe we're the problem.

"But like a light shining in the darkness, God provides seeds of encouragement along the way. He reminds us it is not about us, but about Him, and about Jesus' sacrifice for us all, and that healing comes in His timing.

"Through it all, we were touched by Russell and Marion's faith and positive attitude in the face of terrible news. Our own faiths were put to the test and were ultimately strengthened by Russell's miraculous recovery.

"If this was a test, then they passed it with flying colors. One can only hope we could do the same in the face of a similar crisis.

"One thing is certain: The Lord isn't finished with Russell yet. He has been healed for a purpose. There is more left to do!"

— Chad, Santa Clarita, California

"I was shocked to hear that Russ had bladder cancer. He is probably the most unlikely person I know that would have any major disease like cancer. Russ is very health-conscious, and takes more vitamins than anybody I know!

"*Cancer* is a very scary word, and I immediately sent out prayer requests to people that I knew loved to pray. It was a very difficult season for Russ and Marion.

"It was hard for their friends as well; we love them so much! Praying for Russ's healing jumped to the top of my prayer list. It was comforting to be involved with many of their prayer sessions, and praying with other friends over the phone.

"The atmosphere changed from despair to real hope. The healing was not immediate, but they did a lot of research and completely changed his diet. With time, his skin began to look healthier, which was an indication that he had to be healthier inside too.

"It was an honor and a privilege to witness Russ's healing, and to be a part of his prayer support."

— Jean, Santa Monica, California

"Confession is supposed to be good for the soul, but that's not really my interest in this particular case. The fact is, when Marion first explained Russell's prognosis to me, my mind went to a whole different place than the single-mindedness they both demonstrated for God to heal Russell completely of his cancer.

"And when fellow believers were invited to join them at their home to pray over Russell for a complete healing without any reoccurrence of the disease, I balked and stayed away.

"And though I prayed daily for Russell's healing, the brutal truth as to why I didn't join in communal prayer was that I feared they seemed to be going about the work of prayer without an option that God's will might turn out to be other than our collective desires for healing.

"I'd seen examples of such results in the past, and it threw me for a loop of faith, where I never wanted to kid myself again that enough prayer might change the mind of God.

"But in my Christian immaturity, I missed the point completely. Scripture repeatedly points to our ability to move mountains if we just have enough faith.

If I had joined in with the collective praying over Russell, I'm guessing I would have seen faith in action where I never had before.

"Another fear I had was more of a superstition, that my lack of focused faith might negate or neutralize those who had greater faith, thereby hurting Russell's chances for recovery.

But by not attending, I not only missed an opportunity to demonstrate my love for Russell and Marion—I also whispered to our Savior that I didn't really trust Him.

"I also performed a disservice to both Marion and Russell by not giving them enough credit for having faith or a firm foundation in Christ. I concerned myself too much with how they might be fooling themselves into believing, without a shred of doubt, that God would heal.

"I kept thinking: *But what if it's not God's will to heal in this case… what will it do to their faith?*

"So, there you have it—my confession of doubt. I apologize for all of it. And you need not forgive me. I know you both well enough to know that you already do."

— Don, Burbank, California

"The conversations I had with Russell—when he first found out, and later when he was starting treatment—really moved me. First, I was touched by the irony that someone as healthy as Russ would be impacted by this disease. But what *really* touched me was that Russ was using it all as an opportunity to show how his spiritual health and God were going to be part of this aspect of his life as well.

"I was also touched by Marion's faith and commitment to Russell. Wedding vows are so touching on our wedding day, but they do say 'in sickness and in health.' Marion's love and care for him was a great illustration of how much her vow to her husband and to God meant to her.

"The two of them also allowed others to be part of their journey, so we could see God moving through them, and so others could share in the joys and setbacks along the way. Too often we hide the difficult parts from others and deal with our ordeals in private.

"What a great witness and example the two of them have been."

— Tim, San Diego, California

ADDITIONAL RESOURCES

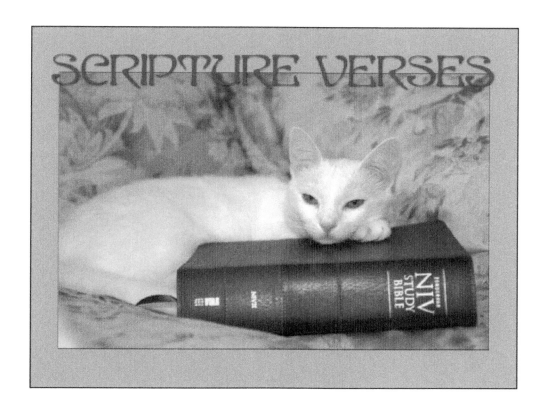

Scripture Verses

OLD TESTAMENT
Exodus 23:25
Deuteronomy 30:19
2 Chronicles 20:1-30
Isaiah 41:10
Isaiah 43:1-2, 19
Isaiah 53:4-5

PSALMS
1:1-3
23:1-6
25:4-5, 12-15
27:1-6
28:6-7
30:1-3, 11-12
33:20-22
34:4, 9-10, 17-18
37:3-4
41:1-3
43:5
50:23
55:22
56:12-13
63:6-8
84:5-7
91:1-16
103:1-5
108:1
112:4-9

116:1-14
118: 5-7
121:1-8
124:1-8
126:5-6
143:8-10

PROVERBS
3:5-6
8:17
10:27
12:14
16:3

NEW TESTAMENT
Matthew 7:7
Matthew 8:5-13
Matthew 17:20
Mark 11:22-25
John 10:10
2 Corinthians 1:9-10
2 Corinthians 10:4-5
Ephesians 5:19
Ephesians 6:10-18
Philippians 4:4, 6-7, 13
Hebrews10:23
James 5:13-15

LIST OF RESOURCES

(IN ALPHABETICAL ORDER)

ARTICLES

Piper, J. (2006). *Don't Waste Your Cancer.* Retrieved July 5, 2012 from http://www.desiringgod.org/resource-library/taste-see-articles/dont-waste-your-cancer

BOOKS ON HEALING

Bollinger, T. (2011) *Cancer, Step Outside the Box.* Infinity 510 Squared Partners.

Campbell, T. C. (2005) *The China Study.* Dallas: BenBella Books.

Contreras, F. & and Kennedy, D. (2001). *Beating Cancer.* Lake Mary: Siloam.

Contreras, F. & Kennedy, D. (2013). *50 Critical Cancer Answers.* Franklin: Authentic Publishers.

Kaufman, D. & Hunt, B. T. (Eds). (2005). *The Fungus Link, An Introduction to Fungal Disease Including the Initial Phase One Diet.* Rockwall: Mediatrition.

Kaufman, D. & Hunt, B. T. (Eds). (2002). *The Germ that Causes Cancer.* Rockwall: Mediatrition.

FAITH, PRAYER AND SPIRITUAL WARFARE

Cooke, G. (2004). *Crafted Prayer.* Grand Rapids: Chosen Books.

Harrison, N. (2001). *Magnificent Prayer.* Grand Rapids: Zondervan.

Hunter, J. (2008). *More Life! Breaking Free from the Spirit of Death.* Los Angeles: Xulon Press.

Lloyd-Jones, D.M. (1976). *The Christian Warfare.* Grand Rapids: Baker Book House.

Kraft, C. H. (1997). *I Give You Authority.* Grand Rapids: Chosen Books.

Moore, B. (2000). *Praying God's Word.* Nashville: B&H Publishing Group.

Osteen, D. (1986). *Healed of Cancer.* Houston: Lakewood Church.

Osteen, J. (1972). *Miracle in Your Mouth.* Houston: John Osteen Publications.

Payne, L. (1994). *Listening Prayer.* Grand Rapids: Baker Books.

Sheets, D. (1996). *Intercessory Prayer.* Ventura: Regal Books.

Siebert, A. (1996). *The Survivor Personality: Why Some People Are Stronger, Smarter, and More Skillful at Handling Life's Difficulties... and How You Can Be, Too.* New York: Berkeley Publishing Group.

Spurgeon, C. (1993). *The Power of Prayer in a Believer's Life.* Lynwood: Emerald Books.

Spurgeon, C. (1993). *Spiritual Warfare in a Believer's Life.* Lynwood: Emerald Books.

TELEVISION AND FILM

Kaufman, D., (Creator/Writer/Producer). (2000). *Know the Cause* (Webcast), USA: Dish TV, Direct TV, Sky Angel.

Wolfson, M. M., (Writer/Director/Editor) (2010) *Vegucated*, (Documentary). United States: Kind Green Planet

Wendel, B. (Creator and Executive Producer), & Fulkerson, L. (Writer/Director) (2011). *Forks Over Knives* (Documentary). United States: Virgil Films.

Kenner, R., (Director), & Kenner, R., Pearlstein, E., Roberts, K. (Writers). (2008). *Food, Inc.* [Documentary]. United States: Magnolia Home Entertainment.

FACILITIES

USC Norris Cancer Center, http://ccnt.hsc.usc.edu

Cancer Center for Hope: http://www.cancercenterforhope.com/

Oasis of Hope: www.oasisofhope.com

MINISTRIES

Embracing Life Ministries, http://www.embracinglife.us

St. Louis Family Church, http://www.slfc.org

Vineyard Christian Fellowship, www.vcfwestside.org

Lake Ave. Church, www.lakeave.org

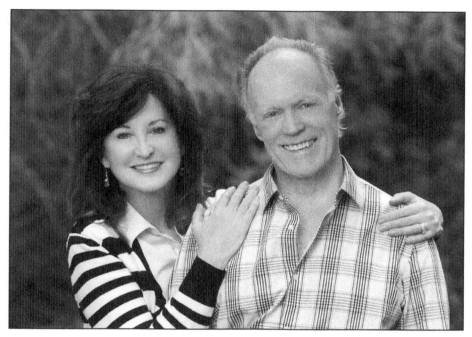

I WILL EXALT YOU, MY GOD THE KING;
I WILL PRAISE YOUR NAME FOREVER AND EVER.
EVERY DAY I WILL PRAISE YOU,
AND EXTOL YOUR NAME FOREVER AND EVER.

- PSALM 145:1-2

Endnotes

1. Siebert, A. (1996). The Survivor Personality: Why Some People Are Stronger, Smarter, and More Skillful at Handling Life's Difficulties... and How You Can Be, Too. New York: Berkeley Publishing Group.

2. Cooke, G. (2004). Crafted Prayer. Grand Rapids: Chosen Books.

3. Kaufman, D. A. (2005). The Fungus Link, An Introduction to Fungal Disease Including the Initial Phase One Diet. Rockwall: Mediatrition.

4. Oasis of Hope. Hyperbaric Oxygen Treatment. (n.d.) Retreived September 26, 2012 from www.oasisofhopeusa.com.

5. Mayo Clinic. Hyperbaric Oxygen Therapy. Retrieved September 26, 2012 from www.mayoclinic.com/health/hyperbaric-oxygen-therapy/my00829.

6. Oasis of Hope. Vitamin C video retrieved September 26, 2012 from www.oasisofhope.com/vitamin-c.php.

7. Oasis of Hope. Vitamin C video retrieved September 26, 2012 from www.oasisofhope.com/vitamin-c.php.

8. Oasis of Hope. Class-IV Laser Therapy retrieved September 27, 2012 from www.oasisofhopeusa.com.

9. Oasis of Hope. Class-IV Laser Therapy retrieved September 27, 2012 from www.oasisofhopeusa.com.

10. Oasis of Hope. Class-IV Laser Therapy retrieved September 27, 2012 from www.oasisofhopeusa.com.

11. PEMF.US. Peer Reviewed Scientific Studies on the Effects of Magnetics on Physical Ailments. Retrieved September 29, 2012 from www.pemf.us/study.html.

12. PEMF.US. Peer Reviewed Scientific Studies on the Effects of Magnetics on Physical Ailments. Retrieved September 29, 2012 from www.pemf.us/study.html.

13. Oasis of Hope. Class-IV Laser Therapy retrieved September 28, 2012 from www.oasisofhopeusa.com.

14. Oasis of Hope. Class-IV Laser Therapy retrieved September 28, 2012 from www.oasisofhopeusa.com.

15. American Cancer Society. Intravesical Therapy for Bladder Cancer retrieved July 9, 2012 from www.cancer.org/cancer/bladdercancer/detailedguide/bladder-cancer-treating-intravesical-therapy.

ADDITIONAL RESOURCES
BY
MARION M. PYLE
FOR

HEALED, HEALTHY AND WHOLE
How We Beat Cancer with Integrative Therapies and Essential Healing Strategies

AUDIO BOOK
Narrated by Marion M. Pyle

HEALTHY, HEALED AND WHOLE PRAYER JOURNAL
Companion piece to the book

HEALTHY, HEALED AND WHOLE
CD OF HEALING SCRIPTURES WITH MUSIC
Narrated by Marion M. Pyle

For More Info Visit:
WWW.HEALEDHEALTHYANDWHOLE.COM

CPSIA information can be obtained at www.ICGtesting.com
Printed in the USA
BVOW10s1148130614

356231BV00004B/8/P